KETO
COPYCAT
RECIPES

Easy, Tasty and Healthy Cookbook for Making Your
Favorite Restaurant Dishes At Home, Losing Weight and
Eating Well Everyday On a Ketogenic Diet

"There are people in the world so hungry, that God cannot appear to them except in the form of bread."

Mahatma Gandhi

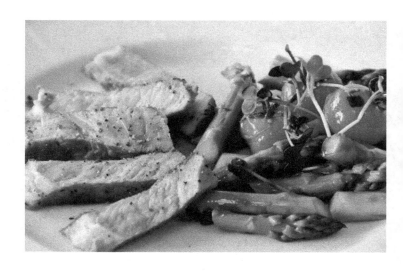

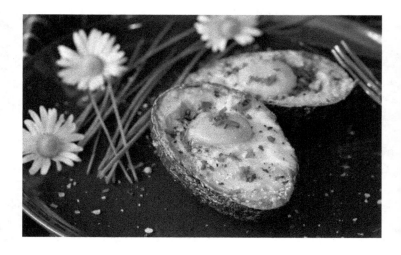

TABLE OF CONTENTS

CHAPTER ONE
INTRODUCTION TO KETO DIET

Ketogenic (just like the Atkins diet) is a term for a low-carb diet. To get more calories from protein and fat and less from carbohydrates, the idea is for you. You cut most of the carbs, such as sugar, soda, pastries, and white bread that are easy to digest.

A ketogenic diet is a low-carbon, high-fat diet, with many health advantages. The diet is ketogenic.

More than 20 studies show that you can help you lose weight and improve your health with this type of diet.

Diabetes, cancer, epilepsy, and Alzheimer's disease may even benefit from Ketogenic diets.

What is a diet that is Ketogenic?

A very low-carb, high-fat diet that shares many similarities to the Atkins and low-carb diets is the Ketogenic diet.

The consumption of carbohydrates must be significantly decreased and replaced by fat. This drop-in of carbohydrate allows the body to become metabolically ketose.

When this arises, the body burns fat for energy amazingly quickly. The fat also becomes ketones in the liver and will provide energy to the brain.

Blood sugar and insulin levels in ketogenic diets will be massively decreased. This, along with improved ketones, has multiple health benefits.

A high-fat low carb diet is included in Keto's diet. The blood sugar and insulin are lowered and the body's metabolism from glucose to fat and ketone is eliminated.

Different Ketogenic Diet Forms

Many variants of the Ketogenic diet exist, including:

Normal Ketogenic (SKD) diet: This diet is deficient in carb, mild in protein, and high in fat. Usually, it contains 75% fat, 20% protein, and just 5% carbohydrates (1 Trusted Source).

Cyclical Ketogenic diet (CKD): This diet requires higher-carb refill times, such as 5 Ketogenic days followed by two high-carb days.

Targeted Ketogenic diet (TKD): This diet makes it easier to add carbohydrates to exercises.

Ketogenic high-protein diet: This is similar to a traditional Ketogenic diet, but requires more protein. Sometimes, the ratio is 60% fat, 35% protein, and 5% carbohydrates.

Only the regular and high-protein Ketogenic diets

have been thoroughly studied, though. More complex approaches are cyclical or targeted Ketogenic diets, mainly used by bodybuilders or athletes.

For the most part, this article's material refers to the traditional Ketogenic diet (SKD), while the other variations still apply several of the same concepts.

Ketogenic diets will assist you in losing weight.

A successful way to lose weight and reduce risk levels for diabetes is a Ketogenic diet.

Evidence indicates that the Ketogenic diet is much preferable to the low-fat diet often prescribed.

Moreover, the diet is so filling that you can lose weight without counting calories or monitoring food consumption.

One research showed that people lose 2.2 times more weight on a Ketogenic diet than those on a low-fat, calories-restricted diet. It also increased the levels of triglycerides and HDL cholesterol.

Another research showed that individuals lose three times more weight on the Ketogenic diet than people prescribed by Diabetes UK on a diet.

There are many reasons for which a Ketogenic diet - including the improved consumption of protein that has multiple advantages as well - is preferable to a low-fat diet.

A crucial function can also be played by increased Ketones, lower blood sugar levels, and enhanced insulin sensitivity.

Diabetes and Prediabetes Ketogenic Diets

Changes in diet, elevated blood sugar, and reduced insulin activity is characterized by diabetes.

A Ketogenic diet can help you shed extra weight, which is closely associated with type 2 diabetes, prediabetes, and metabolic syndrome.

One research showed that a staggering 75 percent increased insulin sensitivity across the Ketogenic diet.

Another research showed that 7 of the 21 subjects avoided taking all diabetes drugs in people with type 2 diabetes.

In yet another analysis, the Ketogenic group lost 24.4 pounds (11.1 kg) relative to the high-carb Group of 15.2 pounds (6.9 kg). When contemplating the relation between weight and type 2 diabetes, this is a significant advantage.

In comparison, 95.2 percent of the Ketogenic group, compared to 62 percent in the higher-carb group, were also able to avoid or decrease diabetes treatment.

Some Keto wellness effects

In reality, the Ketogenic diet began as a method for

the treatment of neurological disorders like epilepsy.

Analysis has now demonstrated that diets can benefit from a complete number of different health conditions:

Heart disease: A Ketogenic diet can enhance risk factors such as body weight, HDL cholesterol, blood pressure, and blood sugar.

Cancer: Actually, a diet is used to treat many forms of cancer and delay tumors' development.

Alzheimer's disease: The Keto diet can reduce and delay the progression of Alzheimer's disease symptoms.

Epilepsy: Evidence has demonstrated that in epileptic children, a Ketogenic diet can induce a massive decrease in seizures.

Parkinson's disease: One study showed that diet helps to enhance Parkinson's disease symptoms.

Polycystic ovary syndrome: The Ketogenic diet may lower the insulin level that may play a key role in polycystic ovary syndrome.

Brain injuries: One animal study showed that the diet would decrease concussions and help recovery after brain injury.

Acne: It may improve acne by lowering insulin

levels and eating less sugar or processed foods.

Meals to Skip

Any food which is high in carbohydrates should be restricted.

Here is a list of foods on a Ketogenic diet that needs to be decreased or eliminated:

- Sugary foods: soda, fruit juice, cake, ice cream, candy, smoothies, etc.
- Grains or starch: products focused on maize, corn, pasta, cereal, etc.
- Fruit: All vegetables, save for tiny portions of strawberry-like berries.
- Peas, kidney beans, lentils, chickpeas, etc. Beans or legumes:
- Potatoes, sweet potatoes, carrots, parsnips, etc. Root vegetables and tubers:
- Low-fat or diet products: highly processed and often high in carbohydrates.
- Some sauces or condiments: These often contain sugar and unhealthy fat.
- Unhealthy fats: Limit your intake of vegetable oils, mayonnaise, etc. processed
- Alcohol: Many alcoholic beverages can kick you out of Ketosis due to their carb content.
- Sugar-free diet foods: often rich in sugar alcohols that can influence the ketone levels in certain situations. These foods are also heavily imported.
- Avoid foods such as grains, sugars, legumes,

rice, potatoes, candy, juice, and even most carb-based fruits.

Foods for Eating

The bulk of your meals should be based around these foods:

- Meat: Red meat, steak, ham, sausage, bacon, turkey, and chicken.
- Fatty fish: salmon, trout, tuna, and mackerel, for example.
- Eggs: Look for entire eggs that are grassy or omega-3.
- Butter and cream: If possible, search for grass-fed produce.
- Cheese: Cheese that has not been processed (cheddar, goat, cream, blue cheese or mozzarella).
- Nuts and seeds: Chia seeds, almonds, walnuts, flax seeds, pumpkin seeds, etc.
- Good oils: Extra virgin olive oil, coconut oil, and avocado oil in specific.
- Avocados: Whole avocados or guacamole, freshly made.
- Most green veggies, tomatoes, onions, peppers, etc. Low-carb veggies:
- Condiments: Salt, pepper, and different beneficial herbs and spices may be used.

It is safer to use a single ingredient for your diet primarily on whole foods. The 44 safe low-carb foods are listed below.

Base foods such as meat, fish, eggs, butter, nuts, healthy oils, avocados, and plenty of low-carb veggies on most of your diet.

Often aim to alternate the vegetables and meat over the long term, as each form offers multiple nutrients and health benefits.

On a Ketogenic diet, you can enjoy a broad range of delicious and healthy meals.

Good Treats from Keto

Here are some balanced, Keto-approved snacks if you get hungry between meals:

- Fatty meat or seafood
- Cheese
- A handful of seeds or nuts
- Cheese with olives
- 1-2 eggs hard-boiled
- 90 percent dark chocolate
- A low-carb milkshake with chocolate powder, almond milk, and nut butter
- Full-fat yogurt with almond butter and cocoa powder mixture.
- Strawberries and cream
- Salsa celery and guacamole

Smaller surplus foods portions

For a Keto diet, perfect foods include meat bits, cheese, olives, scrambled eggs, almonds, and dark chocolate.

Tips on a Ketogenic Diet for Dining Out

Keeping most restaurant meals Keto-friendly when dining out is not very difficult.

Many restaurants serve some dishes based on meat or seafood. Buy this, and substitute extra vegetables for some high-carb food.

Egg-based recipes, including an omelet or eggs and bacon, are also an excellent choice.

Bun-less burgers are another favorite. You may change the fries out for veggies as well. Attach extra avocado, cheese, eggs, or bacon.

You will taste any form of meat with extra cheese, guacamole, salsa, and sour cream at Mexican restaurants.

Ask for a blended cheese board or berries and cream for dessert.

Find a beef-, fish- or egg-based meal while dining out. Instead of carbohydrates or starches, order extra vegetables, and have cheese for dessert.

Side effects and how they should be avoided

While the Ketogenic diet is safe for healthier persons, as the body adapts, there could be some initial side effects.

This is also referred to the Keto flu, and after a few days, it is usually finished.

Low energy and brain activity, elevated appetite, sleep disorders, fatigue, stomach pain, and reduced fitness efficiency are included in a Keto flu.

It would be best to try a typical, low-carb diet for the first few weeks to mitigate this. This will teach your body to burn more fat until you remove carbs entirely.

A Ketogenic diet can also change your body's water and mineral balance, so adding extra salt to your meals or taking mineral supplements can be very helpful..

For nutrients, reduce side effects by taking 3,000-4,000 mg of sodium, 1,000 mg of potassium, and 300 mg of magnesium per day.

In the beginning, at least, it's necessary to eat until you're full and stop too many calories restrictions. Usually, without active calorie limitation, a Ketogenic diet causes weight loss.

A Ketogenic Diet Supplements

While no supplements are needed, some can be beneficial.

MCT oil: MCT oil contains calories and helps raise Ketone levels when applied to beverages or yogurt. On Amazon, take a look at some choices.

Minerals: Due to water and mineral balance changes, added salt and other minerals might be critical when starting.

Caffeine: Caffeine can have energy, fat loss, and efficiency advantages.

Exogenous Ketones: This supplement can help increase Ketone levels in the body.

- Creatine: Creatine provides numerous health and performance benefits. If you are combining a ketogenic diet with exercise, this can help.
- Why: To raise your daily protein intake, use half a scoop of whey protein in shakes or yogurt. There are many tasty products you can find on Amazon.

On a Ketogenic diet, certain supplements can be beneficial. These include Ketones, MCT oil, and exogenous minerals.

Questions Often Asked

Here are some of the most severe issues for ketogenic diets.

1. Can I ever eat carbohydrates again?

Yeah. Yeah. It is necessary, however, to decrease your carb intake drastically initially. You can eat carbs on special occasions after the first 2-3 months; return to the diet immediately afterward.

2. Am I going to lose my muscles?

On any diet, there is a risk of losing some muscle. However, high protein intake and high Ketone levels, mainly if you lift weights, can minimize muscle loss.

3. On a Ketogenic diet, can I develop muscle?

Yeah, but it does not perform as well as on a moderate-carb diet. Read this article for more information on low-carb or Keto diets and workout success.

4. Should I need a refill or carb load? Do I need it?

Oh, no. However, now and then, a couple of higher-calorie days might be helpful.

5. How much should I eat with protein?

Protein should be moderate since insulin levels, and lower Ketones can spike with very high intake. The upper limit is probably around 35 percent of the total calorie intake.

6. What if I am tired, weak, or weary all the time?

You could not be incomplete Ketosis or successfully utilize fats and Ketones. Lower your carb intake to fight this and re-visit the above points. A supplement can also help, such as MCT oil or Ketones.

7. My urine has a fruity scent. Oh, why is that?

Don't be alarmed. This is simply due to the excretion during Ketosis of by-products produced.

8. Smelling my breath. What am I supposed to do?

This is an average side effect. Try flavored drinking water naturally or swallowing sugar-free gum.

9. I've heard that Ketosis is very dangerous. Is it true?

People frequently mistake Ketosis for Ketoacidosis. The former is natural, while the latter only occurs in diabetes that is not controlled.

Ketoacidosis is dangerous, but it is perfectly normal and healthy to have Ketosis on a Ketogenic diet.

10. I have trouble with digestion and diarrhea. What am I supposed to do?

After 3-4 weeks, this common side effect usually passes. Try eating more high-fiber veggies if it persists. Magnesium supplements can also help constipation.

The Ketogenic diet is excellent, but not for everyone

For overweight, diabetic, or looking to improve their metabolic health, a Ketogenic diet can be significant.

It may be less suitable for elite athletes or those wishing to add large amounts of muscle or weight.

As with any diet, if you are consistent and stick with it in the long run, it will only work.

That being said, in nutrition, few things are as proven as the powerful benefits of a Ketogenic diet for health and weight loss.

How This Functions

Eventually, when you eat less than 50 g of carbohydrates a day, your body will be able to exhaust your calories (blood sugar) quickly. Usually, this takes 3 or 4 days. Then you're going to start breaking down fat and protein for nutrition, which will help you lose weight. It's named Ketosis here. It is important to remember that a short-term diet that emphasizes weight loss rather than health benefits is Ketogenic.

Who's using it?

People use a Ketogenic diet more commonly to lose weight, but it can help treat some medical issues, such as epilepsy. Some brain disorders and even acne, people with heart disease can also be supported, but further testing in specific fields needs to be undertaken. To figure out if it's healthy for you to try a Ketogenic diet, speak to your doctor first, particularly if you have type 1 diabetes.

Losing Weight

A Ketogenic diet will help you lose weight in the first 3 to 6 months relative to other diets. This may be that to turn fat into energy, and it requires more calories than it does to turn carbohydrates into energy. It's also likely that you are more comfortable with a high-fat, high-protein diet because you consume less, although that has not been confirmed yet.

The Cancer

Insulin is a chemical to promote the body's food production or use of sugar. Ketogenic diets make you easily burn this food, so you do not have to store it. This suggests that the body requires, and allows, less insulin. These lower levels will help shield you from some forms of cancer or even delay cancer cell growth. More research on this is required, however.

Cardiac Disease

It seems odd that "healthy" cholesterol and lower "poor" cholesterol will be elevated by a diet that calls for more fat, but Ketogenic diets are precisely related. It may be that the reduced insulin levels arising from these diets may inhibit the body from producing more cholesterol. This ensures that you are less likely to experience elevated blood pressure, cardiac disease, hardened arteries, and other heart problems. However, it is unknown how long these results last.

Acne

This skin condition has been related to carbohydrates, so cutting down on them may aid. And the reduction in insulin that can be caused by a Ketogenic diet can also help avoid acne breakouts. (Insulin can induce other hormones that trigger outbreaks to be released by the body.) However, further testing is required to decide just how much effect the diet has on acne.

For diabetes

Low-carb diets tend to be helping to keep the blood pressure lower than most diets and more predictable. But it makes compounds called Ketones as the body burns fat for energy. If you have diabetes, primarily type 1, it will make you sick with so many Ketones in your blood. So it's essential to discuss any changes in your diet with your doctor.

Epilepsy

Since the 1920s, ketogenic diets have also helped regulate seizures triggered by this disease. But again, consulting with your doctor is crucial to find out what's best for you or your kids.

The Diseases

These, as well as the nerves that connect them, affect your brain and spine. Epilepsy is one, but a Ketogenic diet, including Alzheimer's disease, Parkinson's disease, and sleep disturbances, can also benefit some. Scientists are not sure why, but it may be because while it breaks down fat for energy, the Ketones your body produces help shield your brain cells from injury.

Polycystic Disease in Ovary

That is when a woman's ovaries grow larger and small fluid-filled bags form around the eggs. High insulin levels will cause it. Along with other lifestyle improvements, such as exercise and weight loss, Ketogenic diets, which lower the amount of insulin you make and the amount you need, can help treat it.

Practice

A Ketogenic diet can assist endurance athletes as they exercise — for example, runners and cyclists. It helps the muscle-to-fat ratio over time and improves the amount of oxygen that the body can use while it works hard. But although it could aid in preparation, it does not function and other diets for optimum results.

Fast food is impossible to avoid. It is designed to be as enticing as possible, sold using the most modern marketing tactics, and it is everywhere.

For someone who wishes to limit or remove their intake of grains, seed oils, and intensively-farmed meat and vegetables, this makes fast food a minefield.

Yet you do not have to avoid these copycat recipes of Keto fast food.

Your low-carb cake can be had and consumed. Here are some copycat recipes for Keto-friendly, low-carb fast food influenced by McDonald's, KFC, Chick-Fil-A, Chipotle, In-N-Out, Wendys, Starbucks and many others.

Take your fast food copycat recipes with USDA-approved organic beef and chicken to the highest quality (and taste) level. Amazon has some fantastic deals shipped straight to your kitchen with fresh meat.

CHAPTER TWO

RECIPES FOR BREAKFAST

Applebee's COLLAGEN KETO BREAD

INGREDIENTS:

- 1/2 cup of Unflavored Grass-Fed Protein Collagen
- 6 tablespoons of almond flour (see the nut-free replacement recipe notes below)
- 5 pastured chickens, individually divided
- 1 tablespoon unflavored coconut oil liquid
- 1 teaspoon aluminum-free powder for baking
- 1 xanthan gum teaspoon (see alternative recipe notes)
- Pinch of Pink Himalayan Salt
- Optional: stevia squeeze

INSTRUCTIONS:

1. Preheat the oven to 325 ° F.
2. Just the bottom portion of the standard size (1.5 quarts) glass or ceramic loaf dish with coconut oil (or butter or ghee) is generously oiled. Or a piece of parchment paper cut to match the bottom of your plate can be used. It will allow the bread to stick to the sides and remain raised as it cools, not oiling or lining the sides of your plate.

3. Beat the egg whites in a wide bowl until stiff peaks develop. Only put aside.

4. Whisk the dry ingredients in a small bowl and set aside. If you are not a lover of eggs, apply the optional pinch of stevia. Without using sugar to your loaf, it will help offset the taste.

5. Whisk together the wet ingredients (egg yolks and liquid coconut oil) in a small bowl and set aside.

6. To the egg whites, add the dry and the wet ingredients and blend until well blended. It's going to make the batter thick and a bit gooey.

7. Onto the oiled or lined dish, pour the batter of Fridays' and place it in the oven.

8. For 40 minutes, roast. In the oven, the bread will climb considerably.

9. Delete from the oven and cool fully for about 1 to 2 hours. Part of the bread will sink, and that's OK.

10. To release the loaf, loop the sharp edge of a knife along the sides of the dish until the bread is cooled.

11. Cut the slices into 12 slices.

Makes: Twelve slices

NUTRITIONAL (PER SLICE) INFORMATION:

Calories: 77 Calories | 7 g Protein: 7 g | Carbs: 1 g | Fiber: 1 g | Sugar: 0 g | Alcohol sugar: 0gg | Total carbohydrates: 0 g |Fat: 5 g | Saturated Fat: 2 g |

Poly-unsaturated: 0 g | Monounsaturated: 1 g | Trans fat: 0 g | Cholesterol: 77 g | Sodium: 86 mg | Potassium: 51 mg | Vitamin A: 3 percent | Vitamin C: 0 percent | Calcium: 4 percent | Iron: 3 percent

Starbucks's CAULIFLOWER BREAD WITH CRISPY BACON, AVOCADO & POACHED EGGS

INGREDIENTS:

- 2 cups of grated cauliflower
- 1-2 tbsp coconut flour
- 1/2 tsp of salt
- Four eggs
- 1/2 tsp powder with garlic
- 1/2 to 1 Tbsp of psyllium husk
- 3-4 organic, chemical-free bacon slices diced
- 1/4 spring onion, thinly sliced
- 1 avocado

INSTRUCTIONS:

1. To 350F, preheat the oven. Line two baking trays with paper for baking.
2. Toss together 2 cups of rubbed cauliflower, cinnamon, two eggs, and one tablespoon of coconut flour, psyllium, and garlic powder. To thicken, add up to 1 tablespoon more of flour, if necessary.
3. Break the mixture of cauliflower into two. Place each cauliflower blob on one of the lined baking trays and form the mixture into

rectangles using your hands or a spatula. Try not to make them too dense as you want to cook through them, and try not to make them too thin, so they're not going to fall apart.

4. Place them for fifteen minutes in the oven.
5. Test and change the cauliflower toast in the oven. Bake for another 10 minutes, or until baked through and golden brown.
6. To the second baking sheet, add the bacon and spread it out. Place it in the oven and cook until brown is golden.
7. Meanwhile, heat a small saucepan of water and add a splash of apple cider vinegar and a salt sprinkle.
8. Crack two eggs into the broth to poach while the water is boiling. Cook until the whites are thoroughly cooked, and the yolk begins to run slowly.
9. With a slotted spoon, extract them and put them on some paper towel to remove the surplus water.
10. Start plating until the bacon and cauliflower toasts are ready. Place the roasted cauliflower on two plates. Place the poached eggs, crispy bacon, spring onion, and avocado on top of them.
11. Enjoy and serve.

Servings: 2

Nutritional Information (PER SERVING):

498 Calories | 38 g Net fat: | 1121 mg Sodium: | 14 g Carbohydrates: | 8.5 g Dietary Fiber: | Sugar Total: 3.4 g | Proteins: 27 g | 871 mg of potassium

Chili's Chocolate Cake Donuts Classic

Cuisine: American, American
Servings: 8 Servings
Calories: 123 kcal

Components

Doughnuts

- 1/3 cup of coconut flour
- 1/3 cup of Swerve Sweetener
- 3 tbsp powder of cocoa
- 1 tsp powder for baking
- 1/4 tsp of salt
- 4 large eggs
- 1/4 cup of melted butter
- 1/2 tsp extract of vanilla
- 6 tbsp of brewed coffee or water coffee intensifies the taste of chocolate

Glaze:

- 1/4 cup of Swerve Sweetener powdered
- 1 tbsp powder of cocoa
- 1 tbsp of heavy cream
- 1/4 tsp extract of vanilla
- 1 1/2 to 2 teaspoons water

Instructions

Doughnuts:

1. Preheat the oven to 325F and oil it very well with a donut pan.

2. Whisk together the coconut flour, sweetener, chocolate powder, baking powder, and salt in a medium dish. Stir in the eggs, melted butter, and vanilla extract, and then, when well mixed, stir in the cold coffee or water.

3. Between the wells of the donut plate split the batter. You will need to operate in batches if you have a six-well donut tray.

4. Bake until the donuts are set and solid to the touch, for 16 to 20 minutes. Remove and cool for 10 minutes in the tub, then flip out to cool entirely on a wire rack.

Glaze:

1. Whisk the powdered sweetener and cocoa powder together in a medium, shallow dish. To mix, apply the heavy cream and vanilla and whisk.

2. Add ample water before the glaze thins out and, without being too watery, is of a' dippable' consistency.

3. Dip the top of each donut in the ice and leave to sit for 30 minutes or so.

Olive Garden's COFFEE FORMULA

Start to Complete: 5 minutes.

INGREDIENTS:

- 1 cup of Bulletproof brewed coffee
- 1 Tsp. From 2 tbsp. Brain Octane C8 Oil for MCT
- 1 to 2 tbsp. Grass-fed honey, unsalted, or 1-2 tsp. Grass-Ghee's Fed

Start with 1 tsp, if you're new to MCT oil. For several days, then work up to the full serving size.

INSTRUCTIONS:

1. Using Bulletproof coffee beans, brew 1 cup (8-12 ounces) of coffee.
2. To the mixer, add coffee, Brain Octane C8 MCT oil, and butter or ghee.
3. Blend for 20-30 seconds before the latte looks fluffy. Enjoy! Enjoy!

Makes as follows: 1 cup

NUTRITIONAL (1 CUP) INFORMATION:

Calories: 230 Calories: | | Fat: 25 g | Saturated Fat: 2 g | Carbohydrates: 0 g | Protein: 0 g | Fiber: 0 g | Sugar: 0 g | Salt: 0 mg 0 mg

To see what works for you, change the volume of butter, ghee, and MCT oil.

Olive Garden's KETO ICED MATCHA LATTE

Cuisine: American, Japanese
Start to complete: 2 minutes.

INGREDIENTS:

- 1 teaspoon of matcha powder of high quality
- 1/2 Brain Octane Oil tablespoon
- 1/2 teaspoon (or alternative sweetener to taste) stevia powder
- 1 teaspoon of vanilla
- 1 tablespoon of Collagen Protein
- Coconut milk 150 g (or 1 cup), frozen into ice cubes
- 1 cup of water
- 1/2 to 1 teaspoon of the chosen ashwagandha or adaptogenic herb (optional)

INSTRUCTIONS:

1. Connect to a high-powered blender all ingredients except collagen powder. Blitz until absolutely smooth and well-combined.
2. If needed, taste and change the sweetness.
3. To stop unhealthy proteins, apply the collagen mixture gently until just incorporated.
4. Pour over ice and instantly indulge.

Serving: 1

NUTRITIONAL (PER SERVING) INFORMATION:

389 Calories: | | Net Fat: 32 g | Saturated Fat: 28 g | Cholesterol: 0 mg of cholesterol | Sodium: 71 mg | Complete Hydrocarbons: 7.8 g | Fiber: 3 g | Gross sugar content: 0.5 g | Alcohols with sugar: 0 g | Net carbohydrates: 4.8 g | Protein: 24 g | Calcium: 27

mg | Steel: 6 mg of steel | Potassium: 417 mg of potassium

Outback Steakhouse's TURMERIC LATTE

Period for Prep: 5 min.
Complete Duration: 10 min.
Makes: 1 meal, one meal

The ingredients:
- 1/2 cup of coconut milk
- 1/2 cup of water purified
- 1 Tsp. Cinnamon Ceylon
- 1 Tsp. Powder of turmeric

A pepper pinch *
- 1 Tsp. Extract from vanilla
- 1/2 tbsp. Octane Oil Brain
- 1/2 tbsp Butter or ghee fed with grass
- 2 tbsp. Protein Collagen (unflavored or Vanilla)
- The flavor of stevia, xylitol, or monk fruit sweetener
- Add-ins are optional: 1/2 tsp. Powdered ginger, 1/2-1 tbsp. Coconut butter, nutmeg squeeze

Pepper note: Black pepper appears to be incredibly rich in mold toxins, notably aflatoxin and ochratoxin A. A decent pepper grinder with new, high-end black pepper is the best way to do it if you insist on using pepper.

The instructions:

1. In a small cup, heat all the ingredients and then dissolve gelatin entirely.
2. Taste your taste buds and match the sweetness to them.
3. For 30 seconds to 1 minute, dump the mixture into a blender and blitz.
4. Pour your favorite mug into it and enjoy it!

Nutritional Information

Size of serving: 146 g | | 473 Calories | 41.6 g Overall Fat | 36.5 g Sat Fat | 15 mg cholesterol | 18.9 mg sodium | 12.1 g of Gross Carb | 4.2g Sugars | 16.3 g protein | 7 percent vitamin A | 8 percent vitamin C | 8 percent Calcium | Iron 50% Fifty percent

Outback Steakhouse's CBD ROOIBOS LATTE TEA

Start to complete: 6 minutes.

INGREDIENTS:

- 1 cup of water
- 2 packets of Rooibos Tea
- 1 tablespoon of butter or ghee grass or 1/4 cup of coconut milk canned (BPA free)
- 1 Brain Octane Oil teaspoon
- 1 scoop of peptides of collagen
- 1 full CBD oil dropper (about 10 mg, optional)

Optional: extract of liquid monk fruit to taste, ground Ceylon cinnamon

INSTRUCTIONS:

1. Boil sugar, add all tea bags to a cup, and steep it for 5 minutes.
2. Except collagen cut the tea bags and apply the remaining ingredients.
3. In a mixer, pour the mixture and combine until blended. To prevent destroying fragile proteins, add collagen, and mix at the lowest speed until it has just been added.
4. Enjoy being hot, or pour ice over it.

Serving: 1

NUTRITIONAL (PER SERVING) INFORMATION:

Calories: 132 Calories: | | Net Fat: 11 g | Saturated Fat: 8 g | Gross carbohydrates: 2 g | Fiber: 1 g

| Sugars: 0 g 0 g | Net carbohydrates: 1 g | Cholesterol: 0 mg of cholesterol | Protein: 10 g | Potassium: 8 mg

<u>Outback Steakhouse's EGG LATTE COFFEE</u>

Start to complete: 12 minutes.

INGREDIENTS:

- 8 ounces of black coffee
- 1-2 tablespoons of grass-fed butter or 1-2 tablespoons of ghee-fed grass
- 1 teaspoon-2 teaspoon Brain Octane Oil
- 2 eggs raised on pasture

- 1 Vanilla Collagen Protein scoop
- 1/4 teaspoon of Ceylon cinnamon

INSTRUCTIONS:

1. Connect to the blender the eggs, sugar, oil, and cinnamon.
2. Add coffee and blend on high for 45 seconds.
3. Add the collagen protein and mix it for 5 seconds at low speeds.
4. Cinnamon peak.

Serving: 1

NUTRITIONAL (PER SERVING) INFORMATION:

Calories: 3311| Protein: 24 g | Carbohydrates: 4.5 g | Fiber: 0 g | Sugar:0 g | Fat: 25 g | Saturated Fat: 15 g | Polyunsaturated: 2 g | Monounsaturated: 4 g | Trans fat: 0 g | Cholesterol: 402 mg | Sodium: 280 mg | Potassium: 138 mg | Vitamin A: 21 mg | Vitamin C: 0 mg | Calcium: 6 mg | Steel: 10 mg of steel

TGI Fridays's FLUFFY FLOUR ALMOND PALEO PANCAKES

The ingredients:

Blanched almond flour 1 1/2 cups

- 1/2 tsp of baking soda
- 1 tsp (Ceylon preferred) cinnamon
- 1/4 tsp of sea salt
- 3 big pastured chickens, the temperature of the room
- 1/4 cup of pure coconut milk

- Unsalted butter (or coconut oil) 1 tbsp
- 1/8 teaspoon stevia oil
- 2 tsp of pure vanilla extract
- 1/4 teaspoon of apple cider vinegar

The instructions:

1. Over medium heat, preheat the griddle.
2. Place in your blender all of the liquid ingredients, then place all of the dry ingredients on top. Cover and mix to start at low, then increase to high and mix for at least one full minute.
3. Grease the butter (or coconut oil) on the preheated griddle.
4. To shape a silver dollar style pancake (about 3 "in diameter), ladle a spoonful of batter onto the griddle.
5. Once the batter begins bubbling, flip
6. Repeat with the batter before you're done!

Serving: 4

Nutritional (per serving) Information:

Calories: 341 | Protein: 13.25 g | Carbohydrates: 8.5 g | Net carbohydrates: 4 g | Fiber: 4.5 g | Fat: 25.25 g | Saturated Fat: 3.65 g | Polyunsaturated: 5.95 g | Single-unsaturated: 15.75 g | Trans fat: 0 g | Cholesterol: 146.25 mg | Sodium: 94 mg | Potassium: 368 mg | Vitamin A: 346.75 mg | Vitamin C: 0 mg | Calcium: 125.75 mg | Magnesium: 2.1 mg

Red Lobster's WAFFLES OF BUTTERY COCONUT FLOUR

Breakfast Course
10 minutes of Prep Time
Time to Cook: 20 Minutes
Waffles Serving

INGREDIENTS SELF:

- 4 tbsp of flour of coconut
- 5 eggs differentiate whites from yolks
- 4 tbsp stevia granulated
- 1 tsp powder for baking
- 2 tsp extract of vanilla
- 3 tbsp high-fat milk
- 1/2 cup of melted butter

INSTRUCTIONS:

1. Mix the egg yolks, coconut flour, stevia, and baking powder in a dish.
2. Slowly apply the melted butter to the flour mixture and blend well to guarantee smooth consistency.
3. Make sure you mix correctly and add the milk and vanilla to the flour and butter mixture.
4. Whisk the egg whites in another cup until fluffy.
5. Gently fold the spoons into the flour mixture

of the whisked egg whites.

6. Cook until golden brown and dump the mixture into the waffle maker.

Portillo's KETO CREPES WITH STRAWBERRY CHOCOLATE (GLUTEN-FREE, PALEO)

Cuisine American, French
Servings: Two crepes
Components
Concerning Crepes

- 3 eggs
- 3 tablespoons of coconut flour
- I like a stevia blend such as Pyure 1 teaspoon low carb sweetener,
- 1 tablespoon of husk psyllium powder
- 1/3 cup of hot water
- For the Filling
- 1 ounce of dark chocolate
- 1/2 tablespoon of butter or coconut oil
- 1/2 cup strawberries or raspberries (diced)

Instructions

1. In a cup, mix the eggs, coconut flour, sweetener, and psyllium husk powder. Add a little at a time to boiling water, then combine until well-incorporated.

2. Add one tablespoon of oil and turn the heat to medium in a nonstick pan. Add 1/4 to 1/2 of the crepe liquid and cook until the edges

start to brown when the pan is heated. Flip over until golden brown, and allow to cook. It will take approximately 3-5 minutes for each crepe.

3. Put aside the cooked crepe and repeat until you have used up all the dough.

4. When the strawberry chocolate crepe shown above is made, melt the chocolate with butter or coconut oil in the microwave for 30 seconds before it's fully melted. Be careful to stir in bursts, or it can melt the chocolate.

5. Using a pinch of berries and a spoonful of chocolate to line the crepes. Fold the crepe sides to close and fill, if needed, with extra berries and chocolate.

Remarks

Note: When cooking crepes, I recommend using oil in your non-stick pan. Without oil, I tried it, and it did stick a little. Without a nonstick pan, I do not recommend trying this recipe.

Facts about nutrition (per serving):

167 calories, 12 g | total fat, 10 g | total carbohydrates, 5 g | fiber (5 g net carbohydrates), | 7 g protein

Portillo's CHOCOLATE ALMOND BUTTER PALEO CREPES

Cuisine: American
Time to prep: 5 MINS

Time to cook: 20 MINS
Overall time: 25 MINS
Servings: 8 Servings:

INGREDIENTS

Crepes paleo:

- 6 medium-sized eggs
- 1/2 cup full-fat milk from coconut or almond milk
- 4 tbsp of coconut oil melted
- 3 tablespoons coconut flour
- 3 tsp powder of arrowroot
- 1/4 TL of fine sea salt
- 1/2 tsp extract of vanilla
- Ghee (for greasing the pan)

Almond Butter Spread: Paleo Chocolate (Raw Cacao)

- 4 tbsp (either chunky or smooth) unsweetened and unsalted almond butter, Stir-well
- 1 tsp of raw cacao powder (use 1 1/4 tsp for a more pungent taste of bitter chocolate)
- 6 tbsp of full-fat coconut milk from a can (add 1/2 to 1 tbsp of coconut milk per time until desired consistency for thinner batter)
- Small slight sea salt pinch

INSTRUCTIONS

Crepes:

1. In a large mixing bowl, whisk and stir all the

ingredients under "Paleo Crepes" until no lumps exist. For 5 minutes, let the batter sit.

2. Heat one teaspoon of ghee over medium heat in a cast-iron skillet or non-stick skillet. Lower the heat to medium-low when hot, whisk the batter for an additional 10 seconds again.

3. Into the pan, pour 1/4 cup of the batter. Swirl the pan around rapidly and gently so that the batter coats the entire pan evenly. Cook for about 1 minute or until the edges begin to become crisp. Flip carefully and cook for about 30 seconds on the flip side. Switch to a refrigerating rack and repeat the remaining batter.

4. Chocolate (raw cacao) butter with almonds:

5. Combine/stir almond butter, cocoa powder, coconut milk, and a pinch of acceptable sea salt until smooth and creamy. Taste to your liking and adjust.

TAKE NOTE

* After the first crepe, you may have to add additional ghee butter to grate it. As far as possible, add a bit of ghee butter (1/2 to 1/2 tsp.). So much butter is going to make the crepe greasy.

* Optional toppings: fresh fruit or maple syrup for Paleo folks.

NUTRITION INFORMATION

serving: 82 g, calories: 217kcal, carbohydrates: 4 g, protein: 6 g, fat: 20.6 g, saturated fat: 12.5 g, trans fat: 0.1 g, cholesterol: 124 mg, sodium: 168 mg, fiber: 1 g, sugar: 1 g, vitamin a: 200iu, vitamin c: 0.8 mg, calcium: 50 mg, iron: 1.8 mg

Shake Shack's KETO BREAKFAST TACOS WITH BACON AND GUACAMOLE

Cuisine: American, Mexican
Start to finish: 15 minutes.

INGREDIENTS:

- 1 tablespoon Brain Octane Oil
- 2 pasture-raised eggs
- 1 tablespoon grass-fed ghee
- 1 medium organic avocado
- 1/4 teaspoon Himalayan pink salt
- 1/4 cup chopped organic romaine lettuce
- 2 slices cooked pastured bacon
- 3 tablespoons diced cooked organic sweet potatoes
- Optional: garnish of organic micro cilantro

INSTRUCTIONS:

1. Heat a tiny pot to medium heat, then add one ghee cubicle.
2. Crack the middle of the pot with one egg and pierce the yolk.
3. Cook the egg on either side for about 1-2 minutes or until firm, but not overcooked. Take the towel or parchment of a paper-lined sheet from the pot and put on it.

4. Repeat with other eggs. These will be your taco shells.
5. Mash avocado and a table cubicle of Brain Octane Oil and Himalayan pink salt in a shallow cup.

ASSEMBLE:
1. Divide the mixture of avocados randomly and spread half on each shell.
2. Cover every taco with half of the roman lettuce chopped.
3. Put a single slice of bacon on each taco and half of the sweet pommes.
4. Garnish with optional pink Himalayan salt and micro cilantro.
5. Fold in half and eat like a taco.

Serves: 2 (1 taco per serving)

NUTRITIONAL INFORMATION (PER SERVING):

Calories: 387 | Protein: 11g | Carbs: 9g | Fiber: 5g | Net Carbs: 4 g | Sugar: 0 g | Sugar Alcohol:0 g

| Fat: 35g | Saturated Fat: 16g | Polyunsaturated: 3g | Monounsaturated: 10g | Trans fat: 0g

| Cholesterol: 210g | Sodium: 525mg | Potassium: 369mg | Vitamin A: 71 percent | Vitamin C: 11 percent | Calcium: 2 percent | Iron: 9 percent

Shake Shack's PALEO SWEET POTATO HASH WITH BACON

Start to finish: 30 minutes.

INGREDIENTS:

- 1 tablespoon grass-fed ghee, divided
- 2 potatoes sweet, peeled in cubes (about 2 large whole potatoes). 2 cups of sweet potatoes.
- 3 cups sprouts from Brussels, halved with cut outer leaves
- 6 bacon strips, sliced into thick bits
- New rosemary and thyme are sprigs of 2-3
- Cool pink leaves to be decorated
- 2 eggs pastured (elective)

Instructions:

1. On medium heat, heat a large casserole. Add the ghee to the bottle 3/4 teaspoons.
2. Placed in the bowl diced sweet potato and half the thyme and rosemary.
3. Brown gently, all over the sweet potato. Fill in the pan and cover with a splash of water for 8 minutes.
4. Take off the cloth and add 3 minutes of bacon to the saucepan.
5. Apply part of the sprouts of Brussels and other spices.
6. Cook the mixture for about 5 minutes until tender.
7. Top with the remainder of the ghee.
8. If you use, cook eggs as you like. With yolks just set, I cooked my sunny side up.
9. Move the eggs to the platform and dissolve

the peas — salt and serve with the saison.

Serves: 2

NUTRITIONAL INFORMATION (PER SERVING):

Calories: 464.9 | Protein: 29.4g | Total Carbs: 39.2g
| Fiber: 9g | Sugars: 9 g | Net Carbs: 30 g

| Fat: 19g | Saturated Fat: 8.9g | Polyunsaturated:
0.5g | Monounsaturated: 1.9 g | Trans fat: 0g |
Cholesterol: 16.4mg | Sodium: 194.5mg |
Potassium: 964.3mg | Vitamin A: 20157.6mg

| Vitamin C: 115.4mg | Vitamin E: 1.7mg

| Vitamin K: 236.6ug | Calcium: 95.8mg

| Iron: 2.7mg | Zinc: 1mg

Red Robin's KETO LEMON BLUEBERRY MUFFINS

Cuisine: American

Servings: 12 muffins

Components

For Muffins:

- 3 cups (360 g) almond flour (I use 'fine ')
- 1/2 cup butter or ghee (120 ml, melted)
- 3 large eggs, whisked
- 1/3 cup blueberries
- 1 teaspoon (5m) vanilla extract
- 1 tablespoon lemon zest
- Stevia or Monk Fruit sweetener like Lankanto. (Stevia brands vary, so use the conversion chart for your brand subbing for 1/4 cup sugar. If using Lankanto, use 1/4

cup)
- 1 teaspoon (4g) baking soda
- Pinch of sea salt

For Topping:
- 1 Tablespoon (15 ml) coconut oil or butter
- 1/4 cup blueberries
- 1 tablespoon (15 ml) lemon juice, divided
- 1 Tablespoon lemon zest
- 1 Tablespoon lankanto or teaspoon stevia

Instructions
1. Place the oven in the middle of the mixture at 175 C (350 Celsius)
2. Place cupcake liners with parchment paper squares inside the muffin tin or line muffin tin, set aside
3. Melt the butter or ghee in a bowl and blend.
4. Add the almond flour, eggs, vanilla extract, lemon zest, fruit sweetener stevia or Lankanto priest, baking soda, salt, and blend well.
5. Finally, swirl the blueberries softly.
6. Spoon the mixture (up to around 3/4 full) into the muffin tray.
7. Bake until a toothpick comes out clean when inserted into the muffin for 18-20 minutes.
8. Melt the coconut oil or butter in a pan to make the topping, add stevia or lankanto, and then heat the blueberries until they

soften (carefully open them to burst) teaspoon of lemon juice to the mixture.

9. Remove and top each muffin with a little of the topping from the heat. Sprinkle each muffin with lemon zest on top and add a splash of lemon juice on top of each muffin.

CHAPTER THREE

APPETIZERS

Jimmy John's KETO CLOUD BREAD

Cuisine: American

INGREDIENTS

3 At room temperature, giant eggs

Tsp. 1/4. Tartar Cream Kosher salt squeeze
2 oz. Softened cream cheese, softened.
Cloud Bread for pizza

For 1 tbsp. Seasoning Italian
For 2 tbsp. Mozzarella shredded, or Parmesan grated.
Uh. 2 tsp. Paste of Tomatoes

BAGEL CLOUD BREAD

- Tsp. 1/8. Kosher salt, Kosher
- For 1 tsp. Seeds of a poppy
- For 1 tsp. Seeds of sesame
- For 1 tsp. Dried minced garlic
- For 1 tsp. Dried minced onion

Cloud Bread for Ranch
Tsp. 1 1/2. Seasoning powder for the ranch
A third party produces and manages this ingredient shopping module and imports it to this page.

INSTRUCTIONS

For BREAD Pure CLOUD

1. Preheat the oven to 300 ° and use parchment paper to cover a large baking sheet.

2. Separate the yolks from the egg whites into two medium glass containers. Add the tartar cream and salt to the egg whites, then beat until stiff peaks, 2 to 3 minutes, using a hand mixer. Add the cream cheese to the egg yolks, then blend the yolks and cream cheese until mixed, using a hand mixer. Fold the egg yolk mixture carefully into the egg whites.

3. Divide the mixture on a lined baking sheet into eight mounds, spaced them about 4 inches apart—Bake for 25 to 30 minutes before golden.

4. Sprinkle each slice of bread with cheese immediately and bake until melted, for another 2 to 3 minutes. Let yourself cool somewhat.

FOR PIZZA BREAD CLOUD:

1. Apply one tablespoon of Italian seasoning, two tablespoons of sliced mozzarella or grated Parmesan, and two teaspoons of tomato paste to the egg yolk mixture.

BAGEL CLOUD BREAD FOR ALL:

1. Add 1/8 teaspoon of kosher salt, one teaspoon of poppy seeds, one teaspoon of

sesame seeds, one teaspoon of minced dried garlic, and one teaspoon of minced dried onion to the egg yolk mixture. (Or use one tablespoon of bagel seasoning for everything.)

CLOUD BREAD FOR RANCH:

1. Add 11/2 teaspoons of ranch seasoning powder to the egg yolk mixture.

Food (per serving):

50 calories, | 3 g of protein, | 0 g of carbohydrates, | 0 g of fiber, | 0 g of sugar, | 4 g of fat, | 2 g of saturated fat, | 90 mg of sodium

Jimmy John's CHOCOLATE KETO CAKE

INGREDIENTS SELF

To the Cake
Spray for cooking

- 1 1/2 of a c. Almond Flour
- 2/3 of c. Unsweetened powder of cocoa
- 3/4 of c. Flour of coconut
- 1/4 of a c. A meal made of flaxseed
- Uh. 2 tsp. Powder for baking
- Uh. 2 tsp. Soda baking
- For 1 tsp. Kosher salt, Kosher
- 1/2 of a c. Butter (1 stick) softened,
- 3/4 of c Keto-friendly granulated sugar (Swerve, for example)
- 4 Large-sized eggs

For 1 tsp.
- A sample of pure vanilla
- 1 of a c.

The Milk of Almonds
- 1/3 of c. Good coffee that has been brewed Just for the buttercream
- 2 Blocks of cream cheese (8-oz.), softened.
- 1/2 of a c. Butter (1 stick) softened,
- 3/4 of c. Keto-friendly powdered sugar (Swerve, for example)
- 1/2 of a c.

Unsweetened powder of cocoa
- 1/2 of a c.

Flour of coconut
- Tsp. 1/4.

Coffee Instant Powder
- 3/4 of c.

Heavy Cream

1. Place the oven in the middle of a rack and plan to 350 ° c (175 ° C).
2. Place cupcake liners with parchment paper squares inside the muffin tin or line muffin tin, set aside
3. Melt the butter or ghee in a bowl and blend.
4. Add the almond flour, eggs, vanilla extract, lemon zest, fruit sweetener stevia or Lankanto priest, baking soda and salt, and blend well.
5. Finally, swirl the blueberries softly.

6. Spoon the mixture (up to around 3/4 full) into the muffin tray.

7. Bake until a toothpick comes out clean when inserted into the muffin for 18-20 minutes.

8. Melt the coconut oil or butter in a pan to make the topping, add stevia or lankanto, and then heat the blueberries until they soften (carefully open them to burst) teaspoon of lemon juice to the mixture.

9. Remove and top each muffin with a little of the topping from the heat. Sprinkle each muffin with lemon zest on top and add a splash of lemon juice on top of each muffin.

Baja Fresh's CRUNCH CEREAL 2.0 GLUTEN FREE, GRAIN FREE & KETO CINNAMON TOAST CRUNCH 2.0

INGREDIENTS
- 192 g of almond flour
- 2 teaspoons of cinnamon field
- 1/2 cubicle of xanthan gum or 1 tsp of flax meal
- 1/2 tsp of baking soda
- 1/4 teaspoon of kosher salt
- 80 g room temperature grass-fed butter *
- 96 g sweeteners based on golden erythritol or erythritol
- 1 egg

FOR TOPPING ON CINNAMON:

- 28 g melted grass-fed butter
- 2 xylitol or Swerve teaspoons
- 2 teaspoons of cinnamon field

INSTRUCTIONS

1. Preheat the frying pan to 350 ° C, then line two eight-inch parchment then grase cooking spray pots. In a large dish combine the amber meal, chocolate powder, cocoa flour, flaxseed meal, baking soda, and salt.

2. Place the butter and swerve together until it is light and creamy using a hand mixer in another huge bath. Remove the eggs one by one, then apply the vanilla to each other. Place the dry ingredients in a mixture and then mix the milk and coffee.

3. Divide the batter between the prepared pans and bake for 28 minutes until a toothpick inserted in the center comes out clean. Allow it to cool completely.

4. Make the frosting: In a big cup, beat the cream cheese and butter together until creamy, using a hand mixer. Apply the swerve, cocoa powder, coconut flour, and coffee immediately and beat until there are no lumps left. Apply a pinch of salt and milk and pound until mixed.

5. On the serving platter or cake stand, put one cake layer, then spread a dense layer of buttercream on top. Repeat with the

remaining layers of cake, and ice the sides.

6. Store in a refrigerator until ready for serving.

Houlihan's DEVILED EGGS BACON-AVOCADO CAESAR

Start to complete: 20 minutes.

The ingredients:

Eggs

- 2 chickens
- 1 tablespoon mayonnaise
- 1/4 teaspoon of mustard dijon
- 1/8 lemon squeezed
- 1/4 of garlic powder teaspoon (optional; omit if you are allergic to garlic).
- 1/8 teaspoon of pink Himalayan salt
- 1/8 teaspoon of paprika smoked

Filling with Bacon-Avocado

- 1/4 of avocado
- 1 slice of bacon from pasture

Filling instructions:

1. Chop a 1/4-inch slice of bacon and avocado.
2. In a medium-hot pan, add bacon and cook for 3 minutes or until browned.
3. Attach the avocado and cook for another 3 minutes, then reduce the heat to normal.

Eggs Instructions:

4. Carry two quarts to a boil with water. Lower the heat, add the eggs and cook for 8

minutes. (You should also use an instant cooker. Add 1 inch of water to the bottom of the pot, put the rack with the eggs on top of the pot, and set it on the manual for 3 minutes.)

5. For 3 minutes, put the cooked eggs in ice water and then peel and split in half, lengthwise.

6. Remove the yolk from the cut eggs gently and apply the mayonnaise, mustard, lemon, garlic powder, and salt to a food processor and run the processor until the mixture is smooth.

7. Gently spoon the egg white with the bacon-avocado filling. Cover with Caesar egg yolk mixture and sprinkle with smoking paprika, using a spoon, piping bag, or resealable plastic bag with a snipped corner.

Serving: 1 (Per Serving)

Dietary Information:

Calories: 3422 Calories: | Protein: 16g | Carbs: 4g | Fiber: 2g | Sugar: 1g | Fat: 30g | Saturated Fat: 7g | Polyunsaturated: 3g | Monounsaturated: 9g

| Trans fat: 0g | Cholesterol: 400mg Cholesterol:

| Sodium: 650mg | Potassium: 355 mg | Vitamin A: 12mg | Vitamin C: 6mg | Calcium: 6mg | Steel: 12 mg of steel

Houlihan's BACON CHOCOLATE-COVERED

INGREDIENTS:

4-6 slices of healthy, pastured bacon, sliced in half depending on the size,

Up to 1/2 block of dark chocolate of high consistency, melted.

Pink sea salt from the Himalaya, to taste (optional)

INSTRUCTIONS:

1. Preheat your oven to 350F and use baking paper to cover a baking sheet.

2. Place the bacon pieces uniformly on the lined tray when the oven is hot.

3. Place the tray to cook in the oven and make sure you keep an eye on the bacon and check it before you hit the perfect crispiness every 5-10 minutes.

4. Remove it from the oven and gently rinse out the extra fat into a glass jar until the bacon is ready (keep this for your savory cooking). If there is any excess grease, pat the bacon slices with a paper towel.

5. In a little cup or glass container, pour the melted chocolate and start dipping the bacon into the melted chocolate until they're half covered.

6. You can eat it like this instantly, or you can also put the chocolate-coated bacon on a plate lined with baking paper, if you prefer, and replicate the procedure with the rest of

the bacon.

7. Place them in the refrigerator until all the bacon bits are coated in chocolate and allow the chocolate to harden.

8. Take it from the fridge when it's ready and eat it.

9. If desired, sprinkle with a pinch of salt.

Servings: 2

NUTRITIONAL (PER SERVING) INFORMATION:

Calories: 370 calories | Fat: 28g | Protein: 15g | Carbohydrate: 11g | Fiber: 3g | Overall sugar content: 0g | Alcohols with sugar: 4.5g | Net carbohydrates: 3.5g | Sodium: 380mg

Au Bon Pain's BACON CUPS FROM COBB SALAD

The Course: Appetizer

Cuisine: American, American

Servings: 6 cups of porridge

145 kcal Calories:

Components

- 12 slices of thin bacon sliced
- 1 cup of thinly sliced romaine lettuce
- 1/2 cup of roasted chicken chopped
- 1/2 chopped California Avocado
- 1 finely cut hardboiled egg
- 1/4 cup of diced tomato
- 2 tbsp optional crumbled blue cheese

Dressing of preference

Instructions

1. To 425F, preheat the oven. Turn a muffin box of the average size upside down and cover with foil, forming the cups near.

2. Break 6 of the slices of bacon in half. Fill the bottom of each muffin cup with two halves of bacon in an X pattern. Wind a full-length strip of bacon across each cup's edges so that they are sealed with a toothpick.

3. Bake the cups of bacon to your taste until finished. For crispy bacon, I considered this to be around 35 minutes. Remove to cool for 20 minutes, remove the toothpicks to remove the foil from the cups, and turn them right side up.

4. Divide the cups with the salad, chicken, avocado, egg, tomato, and blue cheese.

5. Top-up and serve with your preferred sauce. Or don't dress at all; without it, they're tasty!

Nutritional Information

Bacon Cups from Cobb Salad

- Per Serving Volume (1 cup (as an appetizer))
- 145 Calories from Fat 89 Calories from Fat 89
- Regular Worth Percent*
- 9.9g15 percent Fat
- 1.8g1 percent Carbohydrates

- 0.9g4-percent fiber
- 9.5g19 percent Protein

Maggiano's Little Italy FRIES OF BACON PICKLE

Time of Prep: 8 minutes
Cook Time: Twenty-five minutes
Complete Time: Thirty-three minutes
Portions: 4 Portions
80kcal Calories:

Components
- 4 spears of Dill Pickle
- 8 Bacon Strips, Halved

Instructions
1. Preheat the furnace to 425.
2. Break the spear of each pickle in half, then fifth. (For visual guidance, see above video.)
3. Wrap half a slice of bacon into each pickle quarter.
4. Place a baking sheet over it.
5. Bake for about 20-25 minutes, or until the bacon is crispy.
6. For frying, serve with ranch dressing. (For my favorite ranch recipe, see above.)

Nutritional Information

Serving characteristics: 4Bacon Pickle Fries | Calories: 80kcal | Carbohydrates: 2g | Protein: 5g |

Fat: 7g | Sugar: 1g | Sugar: 1g

Maggiano's Little Italy SHRIMP OF Fried KETO COCONUT WITH CILANTRO LIME DIP

INGREDIENTS:

- 8 wild-caught medium raw shrimp
- 1 egg, pounded
- 3 tablespoons of shredded coconut unsweetened
- 1/2 tablespoon of flour for coconut
- 1 tablespoon of avocado oil

INGREDIENTS OF CILANTRO LIME DIP:

- 1/4 cup of raw cashew, soaked for 4 hours in warm water
- 2 teaspoons of cilantro minced
- 1 lime juice teaspoon
- 1 clove of garlic
- 1/2 teaspoon of Himalayan salt
- 1/8 teaspoon of black pepper, fresh-ground
- 2 cups of water purified

INSTRUCTIONS:

1. Preheat the oven to 300 degrees, then use parchment paper to cover a sheet tray.
2. Mix chocolate and chocolate meal in a tub. Mix together.
3. In the beaten egg, dip one shrimp, then place

it on top of the coconut mixture, spooning more of the mixture over the top to coat. Set it on the lined pan when the shrimp is thoroughly coated in the coconut mixture, and repeat it with the remaining shrimp.

4. Spray or rub the avocado oil on the shrimp very softly.
5. Bake for 20 minutes, or until the surface is bright golden.
6. Flip the shrimp with more avocado oil and spray it.
7. Bake for 20 minutes more, or until softly yellow.
8. When baking shrimp, make a cilantro lime sauce. Drain some water from the cashews, then in a food processor, mix all the dip ingredients and blend until smooth.
9. Serve the soft coconut shrimp on the side with the cilantro lime sauce.

Serving: 1

NUTRITIONAL (PER SERVING) INFORMATION:

Calories: 5999 calories: | Protein: 34g | Total carbohydrates: 14g | Fiber: 6.5g | Sugars: 3.5g Sugars | Net carbohydrates: 7.5g | Fat: 43g | Saturated Fat: 15g | Cholesterol: 262mg Cholesterol: | Sodium: 647 mg | Potassium: 542 mg | Steel: 59% of steel | Calcium: 11%, | Vitamin A: seven percent | Vitamin C: 5%, 5%

Boston Market's SHRIMP OF Fried KETO COCONUT WITH CILANTRO LIME DIP

INGREDIENTS:

- 8 wild-caught medium raw shrimp
- 1 egg, pounded
- 3 tablespoons of shredded coconut unsweetened
- 1/2 tablespoon of flour for coconut
- 1 tablespoon of avocado oil

INGREDIENTS OF CILANTRO LIME DIP:

- 1/4 cup of raw cashew, soaked for 4 hours in warm water
- 2 teaspoons of cilantro minced
- 1 lime juice teaspoon
- 1 clove of garlic
- 1/2 teaspoon of Himalayan salt
- 1/8 teaspoon of black pepper, fresh-ground
- 2 cups of water purified

INSTRUCTIONS:

1. Preheat the oven to 300 degrees, then use parchment paper to cover a sheet tray.
2. In a bowl blend chocolate shredded and chocolate food.
3. In the beaten egg, dip one shrimp, then put it on top of the coconut mixture, spooning more of the mixture over the top to coat. Set it on the lined pan until the shrimp is

thoroughly covered in the coconut mixture, and repeat it with the remaining shrimp.

4. Spray or rub the avocado oil on the shrimp very softly.

5. Bake for 20 minutes, or until the surface is bright golden.

6. Flip the shrimp with more avocado oil and spray it.

7. Bake for 20 minutes more, or until softly yellow.

8. When baking shrimp, make a cilantro lime sauce. Drain some water from the cashews, then in a food processor, mix all the dip ingredients and blend until smooth.

9. Serve the soft coconut shrimp on the side with the cilantro lime sauce.

Serving: 1

NUTRITIONAL (PER SERVING) INFORMATION:

Calories: 5999 calories: | Protein: 34g | Total carbohydrates: 14g | Fiber: 6.5g | Sugars: 3.5g Sugars: | Net carbohydrates: 7.5g | Fat: 43g | Saturated Fat: 15g | Cholesterol: 262mg Cholesterol: | Sodium: 647 mg | Potassium: 542 mg | Steel: 59% of steel | Calcium: 11 percent | Vitamin A: seven percent | Vitamin C: 5%, 5%

Bonefish Grill's QUICK PALEO MEATBALLS BAKED

Start to Finish: 30 minutes (active 10 minutes)

INGREDIENTS:

- 1 1/4 kilos of pastured ground beef
- 2 teaspoons of ghee-fed grass
- 1 tablespoon of vinegar for apple cider
- 1/2 teaspoon of mustard
- 1 salt teaspoon
- 1/2 mild yellow onion, minced
- 2 cloves of garlic, minced
- 1/4 cup of new rosemary, sliced roughly
- Optional: One teaspoon of smashed flakes of red pepper

INSTRUCTIONS:

1. Preheat the oven to 350°C.
2. Place all the meatballs ingredients in a mixing bowl, and when well mixed, use your hands to blend it.
3. Line a parchment baking tray and roll the mixture into small balls, using about just over a tablespoon of mixture per meatball.
4. Bake for 20 minutes or until cooked through, until all the meatballs are wrapped and placed on the parchment.
5. Serve warm or cold and seal in the fridge or freezer in an airtight jar.
6. Servings: 3

NUTRITIONAL (PER SERVING) INFORMATION:

Calories: 474 Calories: 474 | Fat: 21.7g | Salt: 911mgg Salt: | Carbohydrates: 5.6g | Fiber: 2.5g

| Sugar: 0.8g | Total Carbohydrates: 3.1g | Protein: 61.3gg of protein | Cholesterol: 201 mg Cholesterol: | Potassium: 892 mg | Vitamin D: 0mcg | Calcium: 74mg | Steel: 39 mg of steel

California Pizza Kitchen's BUFFALO CHICKEN MEATBALLS INSTANT POT

Components
- 1.5 lb of ground chicken
- 3/4 cup of almond meal
- 1 tsp of sea salt
- 2 minced garlic cloves
- 2 finely sliced green onions
- 2 tbsp ghee
- 6 tbsp of hot sauce
- 4 tbsp of ghee or butter
- Green onions chopped for garnish

Instructions
1. Combine the chicken, almond meal, flour, minced garlic cloves, and green onions in a large dish.
2. To mix it, use your paws, but be careful not to overwork the beef.
3. Using ghee or coconut oil to grease your palms, then form the meat into 1-2 inch large balls.
4. Set the parameters for your Instant Pot to sauté and add 2 tbsp of ghee.
5. Kindly put the chicken meatballs in the

Instant Pot to brown them in batches. Switch them around every minute until they are brown on both sides.

6. Combine the hot sauce and 4 tbsp of butter or ghee when the meatballs are browning and cook them in the microwave or the stovetop until the butter is fully melted. To stir, use a spoon. That's the sauce for buffalo.

7. In the Instant Kettle put all of the browned meatballs and then poured the buffalo sauce uniformly over the meatballs.

8. "Screw the Instant Pot on the lid, make sure the pressure valve is set to "sealing," and then set it to "Poultry.

9. The Instant Pot will beep when the meatballs have finished cooking (about 15-20 minutes). Hit "Cancel" if you are consuming right now, then remove the pressure valve, meaning that your hand is directly from the opening where the steam escapes. If not, for the next 10 hours, the Instant Pot will immediately turn to the 'Hot' setting, and the pressure will steadily decrease on its own.

10. Serve over potatoes, zoodles, and cauliflower rice. Or just eat it alone!

Nutritional Information

- Buffalo Chicken Meatballs Instant Pot
- Quantity Per Meal (1 serving)
- Calories 357 Fat 252 Calories 252 Fat 252

- Regular Worth Percent*
- 28g - 43% fat
- 11g - 69% Saturated Fat
- 130mg - 43% of cholesterol
- 867mg - 38% sodium
- 621mg -18%potassium
- 3g - 1% Carbohydrates
- 1g - 4% fiber
- 23g - 46% Protein
- 300IU - 6% of Vitamin A
- 10.8mg - 13% Vitamin C
- 43mg - 4% Calcium
- 1.6mg - 9% Iron

Cracker Barrel Old Country Store's PALEO NOODLES OF SWEET POTATO WITH THAI MEATBALLS

Start to complete: 30 minutes

INGREDIENTS:

- 8 ounces of braised pork, beef, bison, or venison ground pasture
- 1 tablespoon freshly ground seeds of coriander
- 1 teaspoon of ground ginger
- A few fresh cilantro leaves
- 2 tablespoons of coconut oil or grass-fed ghee, split,
- 2 medium, spiraled sweet potatoes
- 2 tablespoons of amino coconut

- 4 radishes, cut and thinly sliced
- 1 sliced green onion (green portion only)
- 1 lemon or lime, cut into wedges

INSTRUCTIONS:

1. Add the pork, ground cilantro, ginger, and half of the cilantro leaves into a large glass mixing bowl. Mix well into 1 to 1.5-inch meatballs and form them.
2. On medium heat, heat a wide saucepan. Add half of the coconut oil.
3. Attach meatballs to the oven, so that there is space between them. Cook on one side until softly brown, flip and cook again gently. Continue before browning on both ends.
4. Add chocolate oil and spiraled sweet potato to the plate with the meatballs still on the plate.
5. Sauté sweet potato noodles for eight minutes alongside the balls or until the pork is fried and softened.
6. Insert pan and plate noodles.
7. Cover in the pan of cocoon amino. Take the meatballs to coat the plate.
8. Garnish with radish, green onion, and other cilantro on top of nice potato noodles. Over the top spoon some other bowl juice.
9. Savor with salt and eat with a fresh lemon or lime wedge.

Maintenances: 2

NUTRITIONAL INFORMATION (PER SERVING):

Calories: 493.1 | Protein: 23.4g | Carbs: 29.2g | Fiber: 3.9g | Sugar: 8.4g | Net Carbs: 25.2g | Fat: 37.6g | Saturated Fat: 20.2g | Polyunsaturated Fat: 2.4g | Monounsaturated Fat: 11.6g | Trans Fat: 0g | Cholesterol: 81.6mg | Salt: 405mg | Potassium: 763.6mg | Vitamin A: 18451mg | Vitamin C: 3.9mg | Vitamin E: 0.4mg | Vitamin K: 2.4ug | Calcium: 55mg | Iron: 1.8mg | Zinc: 2.9mg

Carrabba's Italian Grill CHILLED PROSCIUTTO-WRAPPED ASPARAGUS ANTIPASTO

Start to Finish: 15-20 minutes

INGREDIENTS:

- 16 large organic spears, rough ends trimmed (about one lbs.).
- 1 4 ounce nitrate and nitrite-free prosciutto thinly sliced box
- Extra virgin olive oil 2 teaspoons of outstanding consistency.
- 1 tablespoon of healthy citrus fruit
- 1 new tea cubicle thyme with just leaves
- 1 new organic tea cuboon with just leaves
- Flaky sea salt 1/4 tea spar and more to finish

INSTRUCTIONS:

1. Steam asparagus for around 8-10 minutes or to crisp, but luminous green. Then dip into an ice bath for about thirty seconds before the process of cooking ends and the spikes are cool to the touch. Gently dry and rinse.

2. You should make your clothes and cook your prosciutto while the asparagus is steaming.

3. Whisk olive oil, lemon juice, thyme, oregano and marine salt together in a small cup, and do not emulsify. Quick whisking is going to do. Just put away. Just put away.

4. First, cut any long part of the prosciutto in the middle in half (not in length). Around eight cuts should be made, so that 16 small squares are created.

5. When the asparagus is finished, wrap around each cooled spurt a piece of prosciutto and put it on a plate.

6. Then dress the plate and apply the sea salt. Add the salt to the plate.

7. Store several days of leftovers wrapped in the fridge. Ideally, if you can keep the dressing individually, it is best. It functions anyway, though.

NUTRITIONAL INFORMATION (PER SERVING):

Calories: 35 | Protein: 2g | Carbs: 1 g | Fiber: .3g | Sugar: 0 g | Alcohol sugar: 0gg | Net Carbs: .7g | Fat: 3g | Saturated Fat: 1g | Poly-unsaturated: 0 g | Monounsaturated: 1 g | Trans fat: 0 g | Cholesterol:

6g | Sodium: 167mg | Potassium: 39mg | Vitamin A: 2 percent | Vitamin C: 6 percent | Calcium: 0 percent | Iron: 2 percent

P.F. Chang's THYME AND FRITTERS LOW-CARB.

Ingredients:

2 medium-sized turquoises, grated.
- Salt 2 tsp.
- 2 tbsp thyme-fresh flooring.
- 1 tsp powder of garlic.
- 3/4 cup of white meal of almond
- 2 eggs organic
- Cooking grass-food ghee

Suggested topping: serve on top, poached egg, premium smoked salmon Suggested salmon

Guidelines:

1. In a tub, apply the rubbed turkey and salt and combine. Put aside 10-15 minutes and let some of the water run out with the salt.

2. Remove the full volume of fluid from the zucchini; you should bring the mixture into a tea towel, squeeze the remaining Fluid out or just use the strainer. Through a bowl and mix in all ingredients.

3. On medium heat, heat a wide skillet. Cover the pan with some ghee and let it melt. After heating the oven, place some of the mixtures on the oven to create a frying pan for a test

lot. Flip the fry softly until the bottom is golden brown. Fry on the other hand before golden brown.4. Slide on a tray the fritter.

4. If the mixture is too dry, blend through another egg (I think these are easier to cook and flip if the mixture is a bit on the runnier side, you would only have to re-mix the raw mix in between cooking the fritters if the liquid starts to separate). Add more almonds before maximum consistency has been achieved if the mixture is too wet.

5. Continue cooking the fritters and, if appropriate, add more ghee to the plate.

6. When they're all ready and fried, the scale starts to start.

7. Serve and savor with your array of toppings.

1. Makes 8-9 cakes with zucchini

Data on Nutrition:

Serving dimensions: 1 fritter | Calories: 1066 calories | Carbohydrate: 4.2 g | Gross sugar: 1.3 g | Fat: 8.9 g | Protein:3.9 g | Fiber: 2 g | Sodium: 50 mg

CHAPTER FOUR

SALADS

Olive Garden's KETO CAESAR SALAD- WITH LOW CARB CROUTONS & CREAMY SAUCE!

Components

- 4 large eggs
- 5 ounces of roughly sliced bacon
- 1 big washed and well-drained Romaine Lettuce
- 2 ounces shaved Parmesan Cheese
- 2 servings Keto Croutons
- 4 Halved anchovies
- 1/3 cup of Keto Caesar Dressing
- Salt to taste
- Freshly flavored Ground Pepper

Instructions

1. Place the eggs and place them over high heat in a small saucepan of hot tap water. Set a timer for 12 minutes until bubbles emerge.

2. Place them under cold water to cool for 10 minutes after the eggs are fried. Then peel and put aside.

3. Place the bacon over a high fire in a frying pan and cook until crispy. Drain and set

aside the extra fat.

4. Place the lettuce in your serving bowl and break it into tiny to medium pieces.

5. Sprinkle with parmesan, croutons, bacon, and anchovies (if the lettuce is used.

6. The boiled eggs are sliced in half and added to the salad.

7. Drizzle with salt and pepper over the dressing and season. To combine the flavors, toss gently.

8. You serve.

Nutritional Information

Calories: 418kcal | Carbohydrates: 3 g | Protein: 20 g | Fat: 35 g | Fat: 11 g | Cholesterol: 255 mg | Sodium: 650 mg | Potassium: 196 mg | Fiber: 1 g | Sugar: 1 g | Vitamin A: 1040IU | Vitamin C: 1 mg | Calcium: 207 mg | Iron: 2 mg | Fiber: 1 g Vitamin A: 1040IU | Vitamin C: 1 mg | Calcium: 207 mg Iron: 2 mg

<u>True Food Kitchen's GREEK SALAD KETO</u>

Components
- 1 Cucumber
- 1 Red Pepper
- 1 Green Pepper
- 1/2 Red Onion
- 4 Feta Cheese ounces
- 1/2 cup of pitted Kalamata Olives
- 1/4 cup of olive oil

- 1 tablespoon Vinegar of Red Wine
- 1 teaspoon of Oregano Dried
- 1/4 teaspoon of Salt
- Black Pepper Pinch

Instructions

1. Halve the cucumber, add it to a large mixing bowl and cut it into slices.
2. Dry and dice the peppers and add them to the dish.
3. The red onion is thinly sliced and added to the dish.
4. Slice the cheese with feta and add it to the dish.
5. The remaining ingredients are added and combine properly.
6. Automatically serve.

Nutritional Information

Serving: 1cup Calories: 226kcal Carbohydrates: 6 g Protein: 5 g Fat: 20 g Saturated fat: 6 g Cholesterol: 25 mg Sodium: 467 mg Potassium: 254 mg Fiber: 2 g Sugar: 5 g Vitamin A: 1215IU Vitamin C: 65.3 mg Calcium: 164 mg Iron: 0.8 mg Vitamin A: 1215IU Vitamin C: 65.3 mg Calcium: 164 mg Iron: 0.8 mg

True Food Kitchen's POKE BOWL KETO SALMON

Components

- 8 ounces of Skinless and Deboned New

Salmon

- Sesame Oil 1 tablespoon
- 1 teaspoon of Sauce Tamari
- Pinch of salt
- 2 Cups of shredded Cabbage
- 4 ounces sliced Cucumber
- 1 tiny Thinly Sliced Radish
- 1/2 Sliced avocado
- 1/4 cup of Cilantro
- Keto Sesame Mayonnaise 2 teaspoons
- 1 Sesame Seeds teaspoon
- 1 teaspoon Black Sesame Seeds

Instructions

1. Cut the salmon into little cubes and placed them in a small bowl.
2. To marinate, add the sesame oil, tamari, and salt and set aside.
3. In two cups, assemble the cabbage, cucumber, radishes, avocado, and cilantro.
4. Drizzle over the sesame mayonnaise, cover with the marinated salmon and scatter with the sesame seeds.
5. Quickly, enjoy.

Nutritional Information

Serving: 1bowl

Calories: 446kcal | Carbohydrates: 11 g | Protein: 26 g | Fat: 34 g | Saturated | Fat: 6 g Cholesterol: 62 mg | Sodium: 236 mg | Potassium: 995 mg |

Fiber: 6 g | Sugar: 3 g Vitamin A: 365IU | Vitamin C: 33 mg | Calcium: 75 mg | Iron: 1.9 mg | Fiber: 6 g | Sugar: 3 g Vitamin A: 365IU | Vitamin C: 33 mg | Calcium: 75 mg Iron: 1.9 mg

Panera Bread's SALAD WITH KETO CHICKEN ZOODLES

Components

- 4 Roughly 1 pound Chicken Thighs
- 2 Cajun Seasoning Teaspoons
- 4 strips of Bacon
- 2 Medium Zucchini Zucchini
- Arugula 4 ounces
- 1 Avocado 1 half-sliced avocado
- 1 ounce sliced Green Olives
- 2 teaspoons low carb mayonnaise mayonnaise
- Two tablespoons of olive oil
- 1 tablespoon of Vinegar Apple Cider
- Salt to taste
- Pepper to taste

Instructions

1. Put the chicken and season with the cajun spice in a tub. Set aside.
2. Over medium-high heat, put a nonstick frying pan, and add the bacon. Saute until crispy, then extract (leaving the grease) from the pan and set aside. Split into bits or crack.

3. Add the chicken to the frying pan and cook on either side for 5-7 minutes in the bacon grease until fully fried. Set to cool aside, then break into strips.

4. Add half the avocado, mayonnaise, one tablespoon oil, vinegar, salt, and pepper to a cup. Blend until creamy with an immersion blender and apply 1-2 teaspoons of water if the dressing is too thick. Only put aside.

5. Spiralize the zucchini and apply the arugula and the remaining tablespoon of olive oil and a pinch of salt to a large mixing cup. Toss them together and split them into four cups.

6. Put some sliced avocado, green olives, bacon, and chicken on each dish.

7. Drizzle and serve over the dressing.

Nutritional Information

Serving: 1bowl

Calories: 533kcal | Carbohydrates: 9 g | Protein: 24 g | Fat: 45 g | Saturated | fat: 11 g Cholesterol: 129 mg | Sodium: 407 mg | Potassium: 880 mg | Fiber: 5 g | Sugar: 4 g | Vitamin A: 1058IU | Vitamin C: 27 mg | Calcium: 80 mg | Iron: 2 mg | Serving: 1bowl Carbohydrates: 9 g | Fiber: 5 g | Sugar: 4 g Vitamin A: 1058IU | Vitamin C: 27 mg | Calcium: 80 mg | Iron: 2 mg

Seasons 52's SMOKED SALMON &

AVOCADO SALAD

Components

- 7 ounces of smoked salmon
- 6-ounce arugula leaves (rocket)
- 1 medium Avocado
- 1 teaspoon of sesame seed
- Sunflower Seeds 2 tablespoons
- 2 teaspoons of Cilantro
- 2 tablespoons of olive oil
- Lemon Juice 1 tablespoon
- 1 pinch of Salt
- 1 pinch of Pepper

Instructions

1. Dice the avocado and mix it in a dish.
2. Add the rocket, coriander, salt, and pepper and toss gently.
3. Drizzle over the lemon juice and olive oil and toss gently.
4. Put it in a serving bowl and add the smoked salmon to the tip.
5. Sprinkle the sesame seeds and the sunflower seeds around them. Enjoy and serve.

Nutritional Information

Serving capacity: 200 g | Calories: 513kcal | Carbohydrates: 12 g | Protein: 27 g | Fat: 43 g Saturated fat: 6 g | Polyunsaturated | fat: 2 g Monounsaturated | fat: 11 g | Cholesterol: 51 mg |

Sodium: 827 mg | Potassium: 699 mg | Sugar: 2 g | Vitamin A: 2100IU | Vitamin C: 36.3 mg | Calcium: 160 mg | Iron: 3.1 mg | Serving capacity: 200 g

Chipotle's SALAD LETTUCE WRAPS WITH KETO EGG AND AVOCADO

Facilities
- Slicer for eggs
- Components
- Fried 4 eggs
- 1 medium Avocado
- Lemon Juice 2 teaspoons
- 3 teaspoons of mayonnaise
- 2 tablespoons of finely minced chives
- 1/2 teaspoons of salt
- 1/4 of a teaspoon of Pepper
- 8 leaves of lettuce or Roman lettuce for babies

Instructions
1. Cut the boiled eggs using a dicing process using an egg slicer. Raise the egg carefully, without separating the slices, first put the egg on its side and slice it. Place the egg on its foundation, add it to a mixing bowl, and cut from top to bottom.
2. Break the avocado into cubes and apply them to the eggs.
3. In a mug, combine the lemon juice, mayonnaise, chives, salt, and pepper and

blend gently.

4. Apply each lettuce leaf to 1/4 cup of the mixture and enjoy.

Nutritional Information

Serving: 65 g Calories: 136kcal Carbohydrates: 0 g Protein: 5 g Fat: 12 g Saturated fat: 2 g Cholesterol: 168 mg Sodium: 419 mg Potassium: 60 mg Sugar: 0 g Vitamin A: 305IU Vitamin C: 1.8 mg Calcium: 25 mg Iron: 0.8 mg Vitamin A: 305IU Vitamin C: 1.8 mg Vitamin C: 0.8 mg Iron: 0.8 mg

El Pollo Loco's EASY LOW CARB SALAD WITH DRESSING WITH PEANUTS

Components

Simple Salad

- 4 cups shredded Chinese cabbage
- 2 cups of bean sprouts
- 1/4 Cup of broken Cilantro leaves
- 4 finely sliced Scallions
- 1 medium diced avocado flesh
- 1 tablespoon toasted sesame seeds

Dressing of peanuts

- 1/3 cup of raw peanut butter
- Lime Juice 3 teaspoons
- 3 tablespoons of water
- 2 teaspoons of tamari
- 2 teaspoons of Erythritol

- 2 tablespoons of sesame oil
- 1/2 tablespoons of powdered garlic
- 1/2 chili powder teaspoons
- 1/4 teaspoon of ground Ginger

Instructions

1. Combine the Chinese cabbage, bean sprouts, cilantro scallions, and avocado in a complete dish. Mix well and break between 4 plates.
2. In a smaller tub, combine all the dressing ingredients and whisk until fully combined. If the dressing is so thick, add a little more water.
3. Drizzle the salads with the sauce, scatter them with sesame seeds and eat.
1. Remarks

Nutritional Information

Calories: 251kcal | Carbohydrates: 13 g | Protein: 9 g | Fat: 19 g | Saturated | Fat: 3 g | Polyunsaturated | Fat: 1 g | Monounsaturated | Fat: 1 g | Sodium: 459 mg | Potassium: 502 mg | Fiber: 6 g | Sugar: 5 g | Vitamin A: 3800IU | Vitamin C: 66 mg | Calcium: 100 mg | Iron: 1.8 mg | Fiber: 6 g | Vitamin A: 3800IU | Vitamin C: 66 mg | Vitamin C: 100 mg | Iron: 1.8 mg

Panda Express's CHINESE CUCUMBER SALAD

Components

- English / Continental 2 big Cucumbers
- 3 cloves of finely chopped garlic
- 1/4 cup of sesame oil
- 2 cups of Vinegar Rice
- 1 tablespoon of Sauce Tamari
- 1 teaspoon of Gold Sukrin
- 1/2 teaspoon ground Sichuan Pepper
- 1/2 teaspoon field Coriander
- 1/2 teaspoon ground cumin
- Salt to taste
- 1 teaspoon toasted Sesame Seeds

Instructions

1. Break the cucumber in half and break it into thick slices. Set it in a wide tub.
2. The remaining ingredients are added and blend properly.
3. Leave it for 3 hours to marinate.
4. Sprinkle the sesame seeds on them and eat them.

Nutritional Information

Calories: 104kcal | Carbohydrates: 3 g | Protein: 1 g | Fat: 9 g | Saturated | Fat: 1 g | Sodium: 170 mg | Potassium: 139 mg | Fiber: 1 g | Sugar: 1 g | Vitamin A: 65IU | Vitamin C: 3.5 mg | Calcium: 19 mg | Iron: 0.5 mg | Vitamin A: 65IU | Vitamin C: 3.5 mg | Calcium: 19 mg | Iron: 0.5 mg

KFC's KETO CHICKEN SALAD

Components

Chicken-Chicken

- 1 pound Boneless Chicken Thighs
- 1/2 tsp of Salt
- 1/2 teaspoon ground Pepper
- 1/4 teaspoon powder with garlic
- 1 tablespoon of Olive Oil

The Salad

- 1 cup diced celery
- 1 tablespoon of finely chopped parsley
- 1/2 cup of Low Carb Mayonnaise
- Salt to taste
- Pepper to taste
- Baby Romaine Lettuce 10 leaves

Instructions

1. Preheat a 200C/390F cooker.
2. Stir the chicken in the mixing dish with salt, pepper, garlic and olive oil.
3. Depending on the thighs' size, put the chicken on a lined cookie sheet and roast for 20-30 minutes.
4. Remove from the oven and set aside for 20 minutes to cool.
5. Break the cooled chicken into small cubes, around 1/2in/1 cm cubes, into small dices.
6. With the diced celery, parsley, and mayonnaise, put the chicken in a mixing

dish. Mix and adjust the seasoning well.

7. Into each lettuce leaf, spoon 1/4 cup chicken salad, eat and enjoy.
1. Remarks

Nutritional Information

Serving: 0.5cup | Calories: 390kcal | Carbohydrates: 3 g | Protein: 16 g | Fat: 35 g Saturated Fat: 7 g | Cholesterol: 98 mg | Sodium: 466 mg | Potassium: 377 mg | Fiber: 2 g | Sugar: 1 g | Vitamin A: 5121IU | Vitamin C: 4 mg | Calcium: 34 mg | Iron: 1 mg Serving: 0.5cup Calories: 390kcal | Carbohydrates: 3 g | Fiber: 2 g Sugar: 1 g | Vitamin A: 5121IU | Vitamin C: 4 mg | Calcium: 34 mg

Popeyes's SALAD KETO TABBOULEH

Components

- 1/2 cup raw Cauliflower Rice
- 1 Seeded and diced tomato
- 3 cloves of finely chopped garlic
- 4 Finely sliced Scallions
- 1 1/2 cup of thinly sliced Parsley
- 1/3 cup finely chopped mint
- Lemon Juice 2 teaspoons
- 1/4 cup of olive oil
- 1/2 Teaspoon of Salt
- 1/4 teaspoon ground Pepper
- Instructions
- In a mixing cup, put all of the ingredients.

Mix thoroughly.

- Set aside for a 5-10 minute infusion of the flavors.
- Just serve.

Nutritional Information

Serving: 2 oz | Calories: 149kcal | Carbohydrates: 5 g | Protein: 2 g | Fat: 14 g Saturated fat: 2 g | Sodium: 315 mg | Potassium: 321 mg | Fiber: 2 g | Sugar: 2 g | Vitamin A: 2430IU | Vitamin C: 50.8 mg | Calcium: 60 mg Iron: 2 mg | Iron: 2 mg | Vitamin A: 2430IU Vitamin C: 50.8 mg | Calcium: 60 mg

Popeyes's CAESAR LOW CARB DRESSING SALAD

Components

- 2 chickens
- Dijon Mustard 1 tbsp
- 1 crushed garlic clove
- 3 Anchovies
- 1 tsp of White Pepper
- 2-3 pinches of salt
- 17 fl.oz of medium flavored olive oil
- 2 oz grated Parmesan cheese
- 1/3 cup of finely chopped Parsley
- Lemon Juice 3 tbsp

Instructions

1. In a food processor, place the eggs, mustard, garlic, anchovies, salt, and pepper and

combine at medium / high speed for 3 minutes or until well blended.

2. Drop the velocity well below medium and very slowly, in a thin stream, apply the oil. It will allow the dressing to break if the oil is used too soon.

3. Attach the parmesan cheese, sliced parsley, and lemon juice and mix until mixed.

4. If needed, taste and change the seasoning. To thin it, apply 2-3 teaspoons of warm water if the dressing is too thick.

5. Serve it drizzled, or use it as a dipping sauce, over your favorite salad.

Remarks

Nutritional Information

Serving: 30 g | Calories: 21kcal | Carbohydrates: 0 g | Protein: 1 g | Fat: 1 g | Saturated fat: 0 g Cholesterol: 14 mg | Sodium: 77 mg | Potassium: 14 mg | Fiber: 0 g | Sugar: 0 g | Vitamin A: 100IU Vitamin C: 1.7 mg | Calcium: 29 mg | Iron: 0.2 mg Sugar: 0 g | Vitamin A: 100IU | Vitamin C: 1.7 mg Calcium: 29 mg Iron: 0.2 mg

CHAPTER FIVE
LUNCH

Subway's FRITTATA KETO WITH NEW SPINACH

Components
- 5 oz. Bacon or chorizo sliced
- 2 tbsp of butter
- 8 oz. New spinach
- 8 eggs
- 1 cup of healthy ice cream
- 5 oz. Cheese shredded
- Salt and pepper

Instructions
1. Oven preheat to 175 ° C (350 ° F). Oven. Grate a ramekin alone or a pan with a 9x9 baker.
2. Freeze the bacon in the butter until soft, medium heat. Then whisk and wilt the spinach. Take the pot off the heat and set it aside.
3. Whisk eggs and milk together and dump them into a bakery or ramekin.
4. Using it in the middle of the oven to add the bacon, spinach and cheese. Bake until fair and golden brown on top for around 25-30

minutes.

Nutritional Information

Per serving | Net carbs: 3 % (4 g) | Fiber: 1 g
| Fat: 81 % (59 g) | Protein: 16 % (27 g) | kcal: 661

Subway's CLASSIC EGGS AND BACON

Components

- 8 eggs
- 5 oz. Sliced pork, in strips

(optional) Cherry tomatoes
New parsley (optional)

Instructions

1. On medium pressure, fried the bacon in a saucepan until crispy. Place yourself on a plate aside. In the tub, leave the made fat.

2. For frying the eggs, use the same pan. Place it over medium heat and break into the bacon grease with your eggs. To prevent splattering of hot oil, you should also split them into a measuring cup and carefully dump them into the tub.

3. Cook your eggs the way you want them. Enable the eggs to fry on one side and cover the pot with a lid so that they are cooked. Flip the eggs for easy-cooked eggs after a few minutes and boil them for a moment. Half the cherry tomatoes and fry them at the same time.

4. Salt to taste and pepper.

Nutritional Information
Per serving | Net carbs: 2 % (1 g) | Fiber: 0 g
| Fat: 75 % (22 g) | Protein: 23 % (15 g) | kcal: 272

Jersey Mike's KETO BLT WITH BREAD CLOUD

Components
- Bread from the Cloud
- 3 eggs
- 4 oz. Cheese with cream cheese
- 1 pinch of salt
- 1/2 tbsp powder of ground psyllium husk
- 1/2 tsp baking powder
- 1/4 tsp tartar cream (optional)

Filling for
- 4 tbsp with mayonnaise
- 5 oz. With pancakes
- 2 oz. Lettuce
- 1 tomato, cut thinly

Bread from the Cloud
1. Preheat the oven to 150oC (300oF).
2. For egg whites in one bowl and egg yolks in another, divide the shells. Remember, as opposed to plastic, egg whites whip best in a metal or ceramic cup.
3. Whip the egg whites along with the salt (and tartar cream, if any) until very stiff, ideally

using a hand-held electric mixer. Without the egg whites shifting, you should be able to flip the cup over.

4. Mix then incorporate cream cheese, psyllium husk, then baking powder.

5. Fold the whites in the combination of egg yolk such that the air stays white in the egg.

6. On a sheet of paper baked bread, put two mixer dollops per serving. The rows are fanized to about 1/2 "(1 cm) thick with a spatula.

7. In the center of the oven, cook until golden for about 25 minutes.

Constructing the BLT

1. On medium-high pressure, cook the bacon in a pan until it is crispy.

2. Set the bits of cloud bread top-side down.

3. On each bread spread the mayonnaise.

4. Between the bread halves, put the lettuce, tomato, and fried bacon in layers.

Nutritional Information

Net carbs: 4 % (7 g) | Fiber: 3 g | Fat: 83 % (65 g) | Protein: 13 % (22 g) | kcal: 705

Jimmy John's SANDWICH FOR KETO BREAKFAST

Components

- 2 teaspoons of oil of canola
- 5 ounces of bulk sausage for breakfast
- 2 oversized eggs
- Cream cheese with 1 1/2 tbsp, at room temperature
- 1 tablespoon of fresh chives finely chopped
- 1 tablespoon of new cilantro, finely chopped
- 1 tablespoon of new parsley finely chopped
- Kosher salt and black pepper, newly roasted
- 1 deli slice of Cheddar Sharp
- 1/4 avocado, sliced into slices of 1/4-inch

Directions

1. In a shallow non-stick pot heat the oil over medium heat. Break the sausage in half with each slice, and create a thin four-inch patty. Place the patties in the pot and cook for approximately 2 minutes, until golden and fried. Drag it to a plate lined with towels of cloth. Set aside the stick and gout.

2. Combine the cream cheese, chives, cilantro, parsley, a pinch of salt, and a few slices of pepper with the eggs.

3. Over medium pressure, pressure the skillet, and the drippings. Add the eggs and stir with a silicone spatula for the first 30 seconds to break up the curds as they cook. Stop

stirring and let the eggs cook for another 30 seconds, then slide the omelet onto a plate (they will still be wet on top). Turn the eggs back into the pan on the uncooked side. In one hand of the shells, top with the Cheddar. Cook for 30 seconds to 1 minute until all eggs are cooked, but still delicate.

4. Placed a "bun" sausage on a plate. Fold the omelet in half, and slide it out on the pot, and then into quarters with the silicone spatula. Slice the avocado with the second "bun" sausage.

Nutritional Information

Calories: 603 | Total Carbs: 7g | Fiber: 3g | Net Carbs: 4g | Protein: 22g | Fat: 54g

Jimmy John's FRIED EGG SANDWICH

Components

- 1 tablespoon ketchup
- 1/2 teaspoon chipotle in adobo sauce
- 2 slices sourdough bread
- 2 slices Cheddar
- 1 tablespoon unsalted butter
- 1 slice bacon, halved
- 1 egg

Directions

1. Combine the chipotle and ketchup and spread the bread in every piece. Put the cheese in an angle between the bread and hang over the sides of the bread. Butter with

half the butter on the outside of a slice of bread. Over medium heat, heat a skillet. Click the buttered-down sandwich. Press until the bread is brown golden and the cheese is melting. Butter with the rest of the butter and flip on the other side (which is facing up). Cook the cheese until they are golden brown. It should take three to four minutes. Remove the heat and hold the sandwich.

2. Meanwhile, cook the bacon for about 5 minutes in a medium-heat pan. Turn the bacon and press two pieces to form a square next to each other. Rub the egg up and cook in the bacon. Continue to cook for about 5 minutes until the egg is set. Slide into the eggs and bacon and open the sandwich (use a spoon to help pull the bread apart). Cut and enjoy, squeeze up.

Nutrition Facts

Per Serving:

386 calories; | protein 16.6g 33% | DV; carbohydrates 28.2g 9% | DV; fat 23g 35% | DV; cholesterol 220.6mg 74% | DV; sodium 969.8mg 39%

Taco Bell's KETO NACHOS BELL PEPPER

Components

*   2 medium bell peppers (a combination of colors preferably)

- Salt of Kosher
- 1 tablespoon oil for vegetables
- 1/4 teaspoon of powdered chili
- 1/4 teaspoon cumin field
- Ground beef 4 ounces (80/20)
- 1 cup full-fat grilled cheese blend from Mexico
- Guacamole 1/4 cup
- 1/4 pico de gallo cup
- 2 teaspoons sour cream full-fat

Directions

1. Break 6ths of the bell peppers through the stem, cut the stem and seeds. In a big microwave safe flavor, add a sparkle of water and a touch of salt. Cover and microwave for about 4 minutes until the pepper bits are pliable. Let cool slightly and then place on a foil-lined baking sheet tightly together, cut sides-up.

2. Meanwhile, over medium-high pressure, pressure the oil in a large nonstick skillet. Add the chili powder and cumin and simmer for about 30 seconds, stirring, until it is fragrant and toasted. Apply the ground beef and 1/4 teaspoon salt and cook until browned and cooked through, about 4 minutes, stirring and breaking into bite-size bits.

3. Have the broiler preheated. Onto each pepper slice, spoon some beef mixture.

Sprinkle with cheese and broil for roughly 1 minute before the cheese melts. Top it with guacamole and pico de gallo dollops. With a little water, thin out the sour cream and drizzle over the nachos.

Nutrition Facts

Per Serving:

390 calories; | protein 6.1g 12% | DV; carbohydrates 47.2g 15% | DV; fat 20.8g 32% | DV; cholesterol 3mg 1% | DV; sodium 624mg 25%

Taco Bell's BLACK AND WHITE BOMBS OF KETO FAT

Components

Slivered almonds in 2 cups

- 1 cup coconut oil, virgin or extra-virgin
- Of your preferred low-carb powdered sweetener, 1 to 2 teaspoons
- 2 teaspoons of vanilla extract free of sugar
- 1 orange teaspoon with a zest
- Small pinch of kosher salt
- 2 teaspoons of cocoa powder unsweetened

Directions

1. Unique facilities:
2. Mini muffin tin with 12 cups; 12 mini liners
1. Line a mini muffin tray with mini liners for 12-cups.

2. In a food processor, pulse the almonds, milk, sweetener, vanilla, zest, and salt until coarsely smooth. Stir in the cocoa powder and remove half of it into a shallow cup.

3. Cover the vanilla mixture with half of the liners and then quickly fill the other half with the chocolate mixture. (A black and white cookie should remind you of that.) Repeat with the leftover combination of vanilla and chocolate. A couple of times, press the tin on the table.

4. Freeze for about 30 minutes until it is strong. If you'd like, you can delete the liners. For up to 5 days, refrigerate in an airtight bag.

3. Nutrition (per serving): 290 calories, 5 g protein, 5 g carbohydrates, 1 g fiber, 2 g sugar, 28 g fat, 16 g saturated fat, 390 mg sodium

Denny's CHEESECAKE WITH LOW FAT

Components

- 9 entire low-fat crackers of cinnamon graham, cut in half
- 2 tablespoons of melted, unsalted butter
- Spray for cooking
- 2 8-ounce bags of cream cheese Neufchatel, softened
- 2 8-ounce fat-free cream cheese containers, softened
- Sugar 1 1/2 cups

- 1 cup of sour cream reduced-fat
- 2 major eggs plus three white eggs
- All-purpose flour for two teaspoons
- Extract 1 teaspoon of vanilla
- 1 teaspoon of finely grated zest of lemon

Assortment of toppings

Directions

1. It is necessary to preheat the oven to 350 degrees F. Pulse the graham crackers into the food processor until they crumble. Add the butter and 1 to 2 teaspoons of water; pulse until moistened. To avoid leaks, wrap the exterior of a 9-inch springform pan with foil. With cooking oil, coat the interior of the pan and press the crumbs onto the rim. Bake for about 8 minutes, until browned. Let it cool for 10 minutes.

2. In the meanwhile, blend all cream cheeses and sugar with a medium-high velocity mixer until creamy, 5 minutes, then mix on low in sour cream. Whisk the three egg whites gently in a cup, then add the two whole eggs, flour, vanilla, and lemon zest to the cheese mixture. Beat until fluffy, 3 minutes, at a medium tempo. Over the crust, pour.

3. Place the cheesecake in a roasting pan and add enough warm water to cover the sides of the springform one-quarter of the way up. Cook for around 1 hour and ten minutes, but still jiggling in the center. Switch off the

oven; keep the cheesecake sealed indoors for 20 minutes.

4. Remove and pass the cake from the water bath to a rack. Run around the edge with a knife, then cool absolutely. Chill before strong, for 8 hours, at least. As needed, top.

Nutrition Information

Serving size: 1 piece | Calories: 188 Fat: 5 g | Saturated fat: 3 g | Carbohydrates: 26 g | Sugar: 23 g | Sodium: 297 mg | Protein: 9 g

Pret A Manger's COCONUT KETO PORRIDGE

Components

- 1 egg, pounded
- 1 tablespoon coconut flour
- 1 pinch of psyllium ground husk powder
- 1 pinch of salt
- 1 oz. Coconut oil or butter
- 4 tbsp cream of coconut

Instructions

1. Combine the egg, coconut flour, psyllium husk powder, and salt in a shallow dish.

2. Melt the butter and coconut milk over low heat. Whisk in the egg mixture gently, mixing until a smooth, dense texture is obtained.

3. Serve with milk or cream containing

coconut. Cover a few fresh or frozen berries with your porridge and enjoy it!

4. Yeah, Tip!
5. Put some into your next smoothie if you find yourself with extra coconut milk. It's going to thicken it up a little to make it deeper to fuller.

Nutritional info

Ketogenic low carb | Per serving 3g | Net carbs: 3 % (4 g) | Fiber: 5 g | Fat: 90 % (48 g) | Protein: 7 % (9 g) | kcal: 481

Pret A Manger's KETO OMELET MUSHROOM

Components

- 3 eggs
- 1 oz. For frying, butter
- 1 oz. Cheese shredded
- 1/4 of yellow onion, chopped
- 4 giant, sliced mushrooms
- Salt and pepper

Instructions

1. Crack the eggs with a sprinkle of salt and pepper into a mixing cup. Using a fork, whisk the eggs until smooth and frothy.
2. Melt the butter, over medium heat, in a frying pan. Transfer to the pan the mushrooms and onion, stirring until tender,

then pour in the vegetables covering the egg mixture.

3. Sprinkle cheese over the egg as the omelet finishes cooking and becomes solid but still has a little raw egg on top.

4. Carefully ease around the omelet's sides using a spatula and then fold it over in two. Take the pot off the fire and drop the omelet on a dish, while the gold-brown turns down.

Nutritional Fact

Per serving | Net carbs: 4 % (5 g) | Fiber: 1 g | Fat: 76 % (44 g) | Protein: 20 % (26 g) | kcal: 517

Jersey Mike's CHEESE GOAT CHEESECAKE

Components

- Crust: -Crust:
- Gingersnap crumbs in 2 cups
- 6 tablespoons melted butter, plus additional pan butter
- Sugar 1/4 cup
- Pinching the salt
- Filling: Filling:
- 2 (8-ounce) cream cheese boxes, at room temperature,
- Log Goat Cheese 1 (12-ounce)
- Creme fraiche or sour cream 12 ounces
- Four eggs
- Uh, 1 cup of sugar
- 2 teaspoons extract of vanilla

- Vanilla Pineapple Compote, according to the recipe
- Unique equipment: 9-inch pan with the springform
- Vanilla Compote with Pineapple:
- Uh, 1 cup of brown sugar
- Water for 1 1/2 cups
- 1 bottle of rum
- 2 vanilla beans, broken, scratched, and reserved seeds
- Juiced lemon, 1/2 lemon
- 1 mature pineapple, extracted top, skin, and heart, sliced into wedges or bite-size

Directions

1. Preheat the oven to 350 degrees F.
2. For the crust to make:
3. In a large tub, stir all of the ingredients together. Butter a plate with a 9-inch springform. Press the crumb mixture on the foundation and nearly halfway up the surface of the tub.
4. For the filling to be made:
5. Beat the cream and goat cheeses until light and creamy in the bowl of an electric stand mixer with the paddle attachment. To mix, add the creme fraiche and beat. Add the whites, once in a while, after each egg has been fully mixed in, pound. Beat in the vanilla and sugar until just mixed.
6. Pour the filling into the crust, which has

been packed. Place them in the preheated oven on a baking sheet and bake for 55 to 60 minutes. Turn the cooking sheet in the center of the cooking process. Tent the springform pan with aluminum foil if the cheesecake continues to color.

7. Take the cheesecake from the oven, and, as it begins to set as it cools, let it cool entirely before serving. Before serving, it is best to refrigerate overnight. Break the cake and serve with Vanilla Pineapple Compote into wedges.

8. Cheesecake, say!

Vanilla Compote with Pineapple:

1. In a saucepan over medium heat, add the brown sugar, water, rum, and vanilla beans. In the pan, squeeze the lemon juice and stir to mix. Bring the pineapple to a boil, apply it, and stir until well mixed. Simmer until the liquid has been diluted, and the pineapple is smooth to a syrupy consistency.

2. Let the goat cheese cheesecake cool and serve as an accessory to yummy desserts!

Nutrition Facts

Per Serving:

267 calories; | protein 5.2g 10% | DV; carbohydrates 22.8g 7% | DV; fat 17.5g 27% | DV; cholesterol 63.9mg 21% | DV; sodium 111.2mg 4%

Burger King's <u>KETO-FRIENDLY DOME LASAGNA</u>

Components

For eight servings

- 3 tablespoons of olive oil
- 1 cup of carrot (110 g), rubbed
- 1 yellow, medium onion, diced
- 2 lb (910 g) ground beef
- 1 and a half oregano teaspoons
- 1/2 cup of red pepper flakes
- Black pepper, for tasting
- 4 garlic cloves, minced
- 1/2 cup of dry (120 mL) red wine
- 28 oz crushed (795 g) tomato, 1 can
- 1/2 cup of fresh basil (20 g), chopped
- Salt, for taste
- 1 broad Savoy cabbage head, divided eaves, and trimmed stems
- 1 egg, pounded
- 2 cups ricotta cheese whole milk (500 g)

Guidelines:

1. Pre-heat the oven to 375 degrees F (190 degrees C).
2. Heat the olive oil in a large pot over low heat. Add carrot, onion and simmer until tender for 8-10 minutes.
3. Fill the beef and the season with oregano, red pepper, and pepper. The beef is divided

with a wooden spoon and cook roughly 10 minutes before browning.

4. Two to three minutes before perfuming, cook the garlic.

5. Deglaze the pot and brown the parts on the bottom of the pot with red wine.

6. Drop the split tomatoes as the wine is halved. Cook until thickened, stirring at intervals, for about 10 minutes.

7. Take the sauce away and let it cool. Mix the basil together.

8. Put a big salted water pot into a boil. Apply cod leaves to the water with tongs to batches work. Cook until the leaves are flexible and smooth, for around 1-2 minutes. Drain well and rinse through the towels.

9. Roll in the refreshed sauce of the beef.

10. On the bottom of the 9-inch (23 cm) round baking plates, put the largest cabbage leaf. Line the open sides of the pan with more cod leaves and rim.

11. Eleven. Spread the beef in one-half of the sauce and spread uniformly. On top of the gravy, dollop 1/4 of the ricotta. Cover with leaves of ice. Repeat it to three more layers with the remainder sauce, ricotta and col.

12. Fold overhanging chops in the middle of the pot.

13. Bake for 1 hour on the center rack of the oven until slightly browned. Enable 20 minutes to cool.

14. Place a plate on the bakery and reverse the chou farci to the plate to eat. Take off the pot, slice and serve on the coils.
15. Have fun!

Components:

- 1 flowers
- Mozzarella cheese sliced for 1 cup (100 g)
- Crème cheese 1 tablespoon
- 1 major egg, struck.
- 1/4 bite of amber meal (30 g).
- 2 garlic cloves, hairy
- 1/2 tea cube of oregano dried
- Thyme dried 1/2 tea cubicle
- 1 cold rosemary teaspoon, minced.
- Salt, flavor
- To taste pepper

Preparation Plans

1. Mix mozzarella and cream cheese in a medium dish. Microwave in 30 seconds, mix until cheese is melted, and the consistency is approximately 1 minute total.
2. Add egg, almond flour, garlic, oregano, thyme, rosemary, salt and pepper, then add to the mixture for a few minutes, to keep them from scratching and stir thoroughly.
3. Oven preheat to 350 / kindergarten (180 / kindergarten). Place in a pastry plate or grate a non-stray paper spray.c.

4. Place the mixture in the bakery. Push securely to one half-1/2-inch (1/2-1 1/4 cm) thick in a sheet even-handled.
5. Bake until golden brown for 10-15 minutes.
6. Serve as you wish: cut into popcorn, cut into breadsticks, or cover your favorite sauce and pizza toppings.

Nutrition Facts

Per Serving: 3

494 calories; protein 38.2g 77% DV; | carbohydrates 38.2g 12% DV; | fat 21.8g 34% DV; | cholesterol 104.5mg 35% DV; | sodium 1625.9mg 65% DV.

Burger King's FLATBREAD KETO-FRIENDLY

Hardee's & Carl's Jr.'s JAZZY CHICKEN FRIED

Components:

- 10 parts
- Hour marinade
- McCormick ® Jazzy Spice Blend 2 tablespoons.
- 1 kosher salt tablespoon
- 2 tea cubicle black pepper freshly ground
- 4 cups (960 mL) of buttermilk;
- 4 lbs bone-in, thighs of the skin-on chicken and blowjob (1,8 kg)
- Pantry
- 1 1/2 kosher salt teaspoons.

- 2 tea cubicle black pepper freshly ground
- McCormick ® Jazzy Spice Blend 2 tablespoons.
- 4 full-fledged cups of meal (500 g)
- Freezing canola oil

Preparation Plans

1. In a big tub, mix the spice blend Jazzy, cinnamon, pepper with buttermilk and whisk.

2. Fill in the marinade with the chicken, throw until fully filled. Refrigerate 8 hours or overnight, wrapped with plastic wrap.

3. Create breading: incorporate salt, pepper, spice mixture of jazzy, and meal and whisk in a large tub.

4. In the meal mixture dip the marinated chicken until fully covered. Move to a bakery or tray.

5. In a large cast-iron skillet heat 1 inch (2 1/2 cm) oil for medium-high heat until 350 ° F (180 ° F) is obtained.

6. Worked in bats, cook the chicken for about 15 minutes, turning periodically until golden brown and the internal temperature hits 165 cents per year (75 cents per year). Place the chicken on a wire panel on a baker to drain.

Nutrition Facts

Per Serving:

887 calories; protein 29.2g 59% DV; | carbohydrates 14.2g 5% DV; | fat 79.6g 123% DV; | cholesterol 102.9mg 34% DV; | sodium 389mg 16% DV.

Hardee's & Carl's Jr.'s SUNDRIED ASPARAGUS AND ROASTED TOMATOES PASTA

Ingredients:

- Medium-sized spaghetti 8 ounces.
- Trimmed 1 pound of asparagus.
- 2 olive oil cucharts.
- Cosher salt and black pepper freshly ground to taste
- 1/2 cup of pesto basil.
- 1/3 cup of sun-dried tomatoes drained in olive oil
- Mozzarella cubes 1/3 cup sliced
- Egg fried, to be eaten

Guidance:

1. Preheat oven to 425 F. Preheat oven. Baked or coated with nonstick spray lightly oil. Lightly oil.
2. Cook pasta according to label instructions in a big pot of boiling salted water; rinse well.

3. Place the spray in one layer on the prepared bakery mat. Dry the olive oil, salt and pepper to taste; kindly mix. Place in the oven and roast for 8-12 minutes, or until soft but crisp. Only let it cool before you break it into 1-inch pieces.
4. In a wide dish mix pasta, asparagus, pesto, sun-dried tomatoes and mozzarella.
5. Serve with a fried egg as soon as required.

Nutrition Facts

Per Serving:

457 calories; protein 16.8g 34% DV; | carbohydrates 66.7g 22% DV; | fat 14.6g 23% DV; | cholesterol 6.2mg 2% DV; | sodium 213.1mg 9% DV.

<u>Jack in the Box's SALAD STEAK FAJITA.</u>

The components:
- 2 olive oil teaspoons, cut.
- 1 ointment, slim cut
- Slimly cut 1 red bell pepper
- 1 orange pepper thinly sliced
- 1 bell of green pepper, fine cut
- 8 Roman cups of salad hacked
- 1 avocado, cut in half, seeded, scratched and sliced finely

For cilantro chalk dressing
- 1 cup of loose, trimmed coriander.
- 1/2 cup of milk with whips.

- 2 mayonnaise ounces
- 2 cloves of garlic.
- 1 lime savory
- Pinch of salt
- Olive oil 1/4 cup
- 2 apple cider teaspoons of vinegar

Due to the steak

- Olive Oil 1/4 cup
- 2 garlic cloves, hairy
- 1 lime savory
- 1 cumin soil tea cuchar.
- 1 teaspoon of chili powder
- 1 teaspoon of preserved oregano
- 1/2 onion tea powder
- Black pepper and casher salt freshly roasted
- Flank steak 2 kg

Guidance:

1. In food processor bowls to make cilantro lime dressing, mix coriander, savory sauce, mayonnaise, ginger, lime juice and salt. In a slow stream apply the olive oil and vinegar to the engine; set aside.

2. Stir olive oil, garlic, lime juice, cumin, chili powder, oregano and onion pulp together in a small cup; season with salt and pepper to taste.

3. In a gallon bag or large tub, mix steak and marinade; marinate, turning, rotate occasionally, for at least 30 minutes. Drain

and cut the steak from the marinade.

4. Fire a medium-high heat one tablespoon of olive oil in a barbecue dish. Work in a lot, cook the steak and toss once, at the optimum temperature, around 3-4 minutes per hand, average rare. Remove from the heat and rest 10 minutes before slicing the grain thinly.

5. Stir in the skillet, applying the onion and roast, until the onion is translucent and gently caramelized, for about 7-8 minutes; leave aside.

6. Heat a tablespoon of olive oil in the skillet. Connect the bell peppers and boil until soft and mildly caramelized for around 8-10 minutes, stirring often; set aside.

7. Into a bowl, put the Roman salad in a large bowl; cover with tomato, pep, steak, and avocado arranged lines.

8. Serve as soon as possible with coriander dressing.

Nutrition Facts

Per Serving:

699 calories; protein 49.8g 100% DV; | carbohydrates 31.3g 10% DV; | fat 42.3g 65% DV; cholesterol 120.6mg 40% DV; | sodium 1450.5mg 58% DV.

Chipotle's BURRITO Easy BOWLES

The components:

- Uncooked 1 cup of rice

- 1 cup of salsa, whether homemade or shopping.
- Three cups hairy Roman lettuce
- 1 can be kernel whole maize (15.25 ounce), drained maize,
- 1 black, drained and rinsed (15-ounce) beans
- Two Roma tomatoes, diced
- 1 avocado, stemmed, peeled and sliced. 1 avocado
- 2 fresh coriander leaves teaspoons
- With the chipotle cream sauce
- 1 sample of milk whipped
- 1 tablespoon paste *
- 1 pinched garlic clove
- 1 lime savory
- Taste 1/4 teaspoon of salt or more

Instructions:

1. To produce a chipotle cream sauce, whisk in sour cream, chipotle paste, garlic, lime juice and salt.
2. Cook the rice in a wide saucepan of 1 1/2 cups of water according to packaging directions and keep it cold and whisk in a salsa.
3. Divide the meal into serving dishes, then top with broccoli, maize, black beans, onions, avocados then cilantro.
4. Serve fast, chipotle milk drizzled in sauce.

Notes:

Two tablespoons of chipotle peppers in adobo sauce can be replaced with chipotle paste.

Nutrition Facts

Per Serving:

638 calories; protein 25.6g 51% DV; | carbohydrates 44.9g 15% DV; | fat 39.1g 60% DV; | cholesterol 244.3mg 81% DV; | sodium 1180.9mg 47% DV.

Smoothie King's VALLE IN FRUIT QUINOA

The components:

- 2 tables of cooked quinoa
- 1 stick, skinned and cut
- Divide in quarters 1 cup of strawberries.
- 1/2 cup of fatty fruit
- 2 pine nuts cups 2
- Hammered mint leaves for garnish
- The Lemon's Vinaigrette
- Olive Oil 1/4 cup
- Apple cider 1/4 cup vinegar
- 1 lemon zest
- 3 tablespoons of fried citrus juice
- 1 sugar tablespoon

Instructions:

1. In a small cup, whisk the olive oil, the cider vinegar, the citrus fruit and the juice with

the sugar to make a vinaigrette; reserve.

2. Combine a large dish of quinoa, an apple, strawberries, blueberries and pine nuts. Drop a lemon vinaigrette.
3. Serve promptly, garnished with mint leaves.

Nutritional Facts

Per Serving:

799 calories; protein 39.8g 80% DV; | carbohydrates 81.9g 26% DV; | fat 36g 55% DV; cholesterol 69.1mg 23% DV; | sodium 1376.1mg 55% DV.

CHAPTER SIX
DINNER

KFC's CHICKEN WITH RED, ORGANIC COLOURATION CETO CHICKEN

Components

Tricolored Roasted Garden

- Springs from 1 pound Brussels.
- 8 ounces. cherry tomatoes
- 8 ounces. Champagne
- 1 teaspoon of salt.
- 1/2 tsp black pepper ground
- 1 tsp rosemary dry
- Olive oil with 1/2 cup.
- Cooked chicken
- 4 breasts of chicken
- One ounce. Butter, to be fried
- 4 ounces. Butter of spices, to serve

Guidelines

1. Preheat to 200 ° C (400 ° F). Preheat. In a baking dish put the entire vegetables.
2. Salt, vinegar, rosemary and more. Pour over olive oil and mix until vegetables are evenly coated.
3. Bake until softly caramelized for twenty minutes, or until the plants.

4. In the meanwhile, rub with salt and pepper the chicken into the olive oil or the butter. Cook until 165 ° F (74 ° C) is applied to a meat thermometer in the larger portion.

Nutrition Facts

Per Serving:

354 calories; protein 27.1g 54% DV; | carbohydrates 23.2g 8% DV; | fat 14.5g 22% DV; | cholesterol 79.5mg 27% DV; | sodium 455.9mg 18% DV.

KFC's CHICKEN SAUCE WITH FETA AND OLIVES KETO PESTO

Components

- 11/2 lbs of boneless chicken thighs.
- Pickle and salt
- 2 tbsp of coconut butter or oil
- 5 tbsp pesto red or pesto green
- Strong whipped cream with 11/4 cups
- 3 ounces. Olives in trap
- 5 ounces. Feta, sliced cheese
- 1 fine chopped clove of garlic.
- To represent
- 5 ounces. Greens leafy
- Olive oil 4 tbsp
- Salt and black pepper ground

Guidelines

1. Preheat to 200 ° C (400 ° F). Preheat.

2. Break the chicken to bits in bite — salt and pepper season.

3. To a large pot, add butter or oil, and then stir in batches at medium to high heat to golden brown chicken bits.

4. Mix the pesto with heavy cream into a cup, using the store-bought low-carb, red or green pesto.

5. Place the fried chicken parts with olives, feta and garlic in a bakery bowl. Add the combination of pesto and milk.

6. Bake 20-30 minutes in an oven, until the dish bubbly rotates around its edges, and bright brown.

Nutrition Facts

Per Serving:

370 calories; protein 26.5g 54% DV; | carbohydrates 25g 8% DV; | fat 15.5g 28% DV; | cholesterol 79.5mg 27% DV; | sodium 455.9mg 18% DV.

Buffalo Wild Wings's KETO CHICKEN SKEWERS AND DIP

Components

Skewers of chicken
- four-eight skewers of wood
- 4 breasts of chicken
- Salt 1/2 tsp.
- 1/4 tsp black potato field

- Olive oil 2 tbsp.

Spinach spinach dip

- 2 slices of medium olive oil.
- 2 ounces. Spinach frozen, cut
- Dry parsley with 2 tbsp
- Dill 1 tbsp 1 tbsp
- Powder with 1 tsp onion.
- Salt 1/2 tsp.
- 1/4 tsp black potato field
- 1 mayonnaise cup
- Sour cream with 4 tbsp
- 2 tsp citrus fruits.

Fries with root celery

- 1 lb root of celery
- Olive oil 2 tbsp.
- Salt 1/2 tsp.
- 1/4 tsp black potato field

Guidelines

- Just dip the dip. Thaw and drain extra water from the thaw frozen spinach. Put the other ingredients in a bowl, and combine well.
- Let the fried and skewers sit as you prepare them in the refrigerator.
- Using the broil oven setting, ideally preheat the oven to 400 ° F (200 ° C).
- Break the chicken into 1-inch pieces and place it in a bowl or bag of plastic.
- Add oil and herbs, blend together. Marinate for 5–10 minutes at room temperature. In

the meantime, cook the fries according to step 9.

- Thread of chicken parts 4 or 8 smaller skewers. Place it in a paper bakery parchment.
- Cook with the chicken for 20-30 minutes or to cook thoroughly. Set the time according to distance. Keep warm as long as the fries are finished.
- If you have a convection oven, you can cook fries and skewers concurrently. However, note that frying could be appropriate for a little shorter baking time.
- Peel and cut into strips the celery root. Place it in a bowl or bag of plastic. Season and add oil with salt and pepper. Shake or stir. Just stir.
- Spread out on a baker or in a wide tub. Bake until golden and soft for 20 minutes.

Nutritional Facts

Per Serving:

441 calories; protein 42.4g 85% DV; | carbohydrates 21.3g 7% DV; | fat 20.2g 31% DV; | cholesterol 118.3mg 39% DV; | sodium 402.1mg 16% DV.

Cracker Barrel Old Country Store's SPREE AND FREE TO HAMBURGERS BRUSSELS

Components:

- 1 pound of bovine soil
- Bacon, diced 1/2 lb
- Split in half 1 pound Brussels
- Sour cream with 4 tbsp.
- 2 ounces. Butter Butter
- 5 ounces. Shredding of cheese
- 1 Italian seasoning tablespoon
- Salt and potato

Guidelines

1. Place the furnace at 425 ° F (220 ° C).
2. Brush with butter the bacon and sprouts. Season and add savory cream. Place it in a baking dish.
3. Fry the gold-brown soil beef and scatter with the sprouts on top, season with salt and pepper. Add herbs and forage. Add them.
4. Set in the middle of the oven for 15 minutes or until cooked. You should serve a fresh salad and even a dollop of mayonnaise.

Nutritional Facts

Per Serving:

401 calories; protein 20.3g 41% DV; carbohydrates 32.9g 11% DV; fat 19.4g 30% DV; cholesterol 68.3mg 23% DV; sodium 768.5mg 31% DV.

Outback Steakhouse's KETO STIR-FRY ASIAN STIR-FRY

Components:

- 11/2 lbs green cod
- 4 ounces. Butter, pause Butter
- Salt 1 tsp.
- 1 TL of powdered onion
- 1/2 TL of black pepper field
- 1 dough with white wine vinegar
- 2 garlic cloves, hairy
- Chili's 1 tsp flakes
- 1 tbsp of ginger young, fine-cut or grated
- 11/4 pounds of beef dirt.
- 3 skulls, sliced into slices of 1/2 inch
- 1 sésame oil table cubicle.
- Crazy Mayonnaise
- 1 mayonnaise cup
- 1/2 tbsp of wasabi paste

Guidelines

1. The cod is finely shredded using a sharp knife or food processor.
2. In a large pot or wok pot, fry the coco in half of the butter over medium-high heat. The col took a while to smooth, but let it not turn brown.
3. Adding spices and vinegar. Remove and cook a few minutes longer. Put the chicken in a cup.

4. Melt the rest of the butter in the same frying pan. In addition to the garlic, chili and ginger. For a few minutes, saute.
5. When the beef is thoroughly cold, replace ground and brown meat once a large proportion of the juices have evaporated. Heat a lot lower.
6. Add scallions and chocolate to the beef. Mix until everything is hot – salt and pepper to taste. Sprinkle with sesame oil before serving.
7. Mix wasabi mayonnaise in the starting with a little wasabi and adding more until the seasoning is right. Eat the stir-fry warmly with a bowl of wasabi mayonnaise.

Nutritional Facts

Per Serving:

61 calories; protein 0.8g 2% DV; | carbohydrates 13.8g 4% DV; | fat 0.1g; | cholesterol 1.1mg; | sodium 720.3mg 29% DV.

Olive Garden's ASIAN FROM THAI BASIL SAUCE FROM KETO

Components

Meatballs
- Field of 11/4 lb pork
- 1/2 onion yellow, hacked
- 1 fresh ginger tablespoon, grilled
- 1 tbsp tuna sauce

- Black ground of 1 tsp of pepper
- Butter or cocoa oil four tablespoons.
- 11/4 lbs of green chopped chip.
- 2 ounces. Coconut oil or butter
- Onion Salad Pickled
- One ounce. Scallions, cut thinly
- 1 tbsp vinegar of rice
- 2 tbsp of water
- 1/2 tsp of salt
- One pepper of red chili, thinly sliced
- Basil sauce from Thailand
- 2 ounces. Radishes, minced radishes
- 3/4 cup of mayonnaise
- Salt and potato
- 1 tbsp of fresh Thai basil, finely chopped

Guidelines

1. Preheat the oven to 100 ° C (° F).
2. Onion Salad Pickled
3. For the pickled onion salad, slice the chili pepper and scallions. In a small tub, mix the rice vinegar, water, and salt. Attach the chili and scallions and leave for 5-10 minutes to put aside.
4. Basil sauce from Thailand
5. Finely cut the radishes and blend them with Thai basil and mayonnaise. To taste, add salt and pepper. Reserve. Reserve.
6. Meatballs Meatballs
7. Mix all the recipes for the meatball. "Form

into 1" balls using wet hands, which should take between 30-34 balls.

8. Fried meatballs in oil or butter on medium heat until thoroughly fried and golden brown. Switch to an oven-proof dish and keep the oven warm.

9. Raise the heat to medium-high using the same pan. Add the shredded cabbage and stir regularly until the cabbage is browned, but still a little chewy — season with salt and pepper.

10. Plate the cabbage on top of the meatballs and serve on the side with the sauce and pickled onions.

Nutrition Facts

Per Serving:

715 calories; protein 49.8g 100% DV; | carbohydrates 58.6g 19% DV; | fat 30g 46% DV; | cholesterol 155.9mg 52% DV; | sodium 1181.9mg 47% DV.

Applebee's KOHLSLAW KETO

Components: Components
- 1 pound of kohlrabis
- 1 cup of mayonnaise or vegan mayonnaise
- Salt and potato
- New parsley (optional)

Guidelines
- Strip the kohlrabi. Make sure that all rough,

woody bits are cut off. Finely shave, slice, and shred it and put it in a tub.

- Add the mayonnaise and optional fresh herbs. To taste, add salt and pepper.

Nutrition Facts

Per Serving:

442 calories; protein 46.5g 93% DV; | carbohydrates 5.8g 2% DV; | fat 25.3g 39% DV; | cholesterol 216.8mg 72% DV; | sodium 1604.7mg 64% DV.

Starbucks's COLESLAW WITH MIXED CABBAGE

Components
- Green cabbage 8 oz.
- 4 ounces of red cabbage
- 4 ounces of kale
- 1 mayonnaise cup
- 1/2 tsp of salt
- 1/2 TL of black pepper field

Guidelines
1. With a strong knife, mandolin slicer, or a food processor, split the cabbage.
2. Place the mayonnaise, salt, and pepper in a bowl and add them. Stir well and leave to rest for ten minutes.

Nutrition Facts

Per Serving:

632 calories; protein 9.2g 18% DV; | carbohydrates 39.8g 13% DV; | fat 51.3g 79% DV; | cholesterol 27.1mg 9% DV; | sodium 652.5mg 26% DV.

Starbucks's MEAT PIE FROM KETO

Components

Crust of pie

- 3/4 cup of almond flour
- 4 tbsp of sesame seeds
- 4 tbsp of flour of coconut
- 1 tbsp powder of ground psyllium husk
- 1 tsp powder for baking
- 1 pinch of salt

Olive oil or coconut oil 3 tbsp, melted

- 1 egg
- 4 tbsp of water

Topping With

- 8 ounces of cottage cheese
- 7 oz. shredding of cheese

Filling for

- 1/2 yellow onion, finely chopped
- 1 fine chopped clove of garlic.
- 2 tablespoons of butter or olive oil
- 11/4 lbs ground beef or ground lamb
- 1 tbsp of dried oregano or basil dried
- Salt and potato
- Tomato paste or ajvar relish 4 tbsp

- 1/2 cup of water

Instructions

1. Preheat the oven to 175 ° C (350 ° F).

2. In butter or olive oil, cook onion and garlic over medium heat for a few minutes, until the onion is tender. Add ground beef and keep frying. Add oregano or basil. To taste salt and pepper.

3. Add tomato paste or ajvar relish. Add water. Lower the heat and cook for at least 20 minutes. Make the dough for the crust as the meat simmers.

4. In a food processor, combine all the crust components for a few minutes before the dough turns into a ball. You should mix with a fork by hand if you don't have a food processor.

5. To make it easy to extract the pie until it is finished, place a circular piece of parchment paper in a well-greased springform pan or deep-dish pie pan, 9-10 inches (23-25 cm) in diameter. Spread the dough in the pan and out along the sides. Use a spatula or well-greased fingers. Pinch the bottom of the crust with a fork until the crust is baked into the pan.

6. For 10-15 minutes, pre-bake the crust. Remove from the oven and put the meat in the crust. Blend the cottage cheese and shredded cheese, and layer on top of the pie.

7. Bake for 30-40 minutes on the lower rack or

until the pie has become a golden color.

Nutrition Facts

Per Serving:

424 calories; protein 30.4g 61% DV; | carbohydrates 14.9g 5% DV; | fat 26.8g 41% DV; | cholesterol 117.4mg 39% DV; | sodium 1426.6mg 57% DV.

In-N-Out Burger's CLASSIC KETO HAMBURGER

Components

Keto hamburger buns

- 1¼ cups super fine almond flour
- 5 tbsp ground psyllium husk powder
- 2 tsp baking powder
- 1 tsp sea salt
- 1¼ cups water
- 2 tsp white wine vinegar or cider vinegar
- 3 egg whites
- 1 tbsp sesame seeds

Hamburger

- 1¾ lbs ground beef
- 1 oz. butter or olive oil, for frying
- Salt and pepper
- 2 oz. lettuce, shredded
- 1 tomato, cut thinly
- 1 red onion, sliced thinly

- 1/2 cup of mayonnaise
- 5 oz. With pancakes

Instructions

Buns from Keto

1. Preheat the oven to 175 ° C (350 ° F).
2. Start by making the buns for the hamburger. Mix the dried ingredients in a bowl.
3. Carry to a boil with water. When beating with a hand mixer for about 30 seconds, add the sugar, the vinegar, and the egg whites to the dish. Don't overmix the dough; it can imitate Play-Doh inconsistency.
4. Shape the dough into separate pieces of bread, one for each serving, with moist hands. Sprinkle on top of sesame seeds. Make sure to leave enough space for the buns to double in size on the baking sheet.
5. Bake in the oven for 50-60 minutes on the lower shelf. By touching the bottom of the buns, they're done until you hear a hollow echo.

Hamburger

1. Over medium heat, cook the strips of bacon.
2. Either grill or fry the ground beef into individual hamburgers. When the hamburgers are almost cooked, season with salt and pepper.
3. Break each roll in half and spread on each half a generous amount of mayonnaise.
4. Create the hamburger according to your

preference.

5. Pair for extra crunch with a side of coleslaw!

Nutrition Facts

Per Serving:

350 calories; protein 20.6g 41% DV; | carbohydrates 12g 4% DV; | fat 24g 37% DV; | cholesterol 74.9mg 25% DV; | sodium 694.1mg 28% DV.

In-N-Out Burger's KETO GOAT CHEESEBURGER AND FRIES AND ZUCCHINI

Components

Spicy Mayonnaise with Tomato
- 1 cup of mayonnaise
- 1 tablespoon tomato paste
- 1 cayenne pepper poke
- Salt and pepper

Fries with zucchini
- 1 zucchini
- 11/3 cups of almond flour
- 11/3 cups parmesan cheese grated
- 1 TL of onion powder
- 1 tsp of salt
- 1/2 tsp of pepper
- 2 chickens
- 3 tablespoons olive oil

Hamburger

- 1 oz. Olive Oil or Butter
- 2 red onions
- 1 tbsp vinegar for red wine
- Ground beef 11/2 lbs
- Salt and pepper
- 4 oz. Cheese Goat Cheese
- 3 oz. Lettuce Lettuce

Instructions

- Preheat the furnace to 200 ° C (400 ° F).
- Both the tomato mayo ingredients are combined and put aside in the refrigerator.
- Line the parchment paper with a baking sheet.
- Drop the seeds and cut the zucchini lengthwise. Divide into sticks, about 1/4 to 1/2 inch diameter.
- In a tub, smash the eggs and whisk to mix.
- On a pan, add together the almond flour, parmesan cheese, onion powder, salt, and pepper.
- In the flour mixture, throw the rods and dip each rod in the eggs to coat them. Finish it with another flour coating.
- On the baking sheet put the fries and drizzle the olive oil on top—Bake for 20-25 minutes or until golden brown in the oven.
- In the meantime, get the burgers ready. Thinly slice the onions and sauté in the butter until tender over medium heat. Towards the top, add the vinegar, add a

swirl, and minimize until smooth. To taste, apply salt and pepper. Put aside to serve.

- Oh. 10. Shape the burger patties and fry them to your liking, or grill them. With salt and pepper, season.
- 11. Place the burgers and the onion mixture on beds of lettuce. Serve with zucchini fries and spicy tomato mayo and place the goat cheese on top.

Nutrition Facts

Per Serving: 350 calories; protein 20.6g 41% DV; | carbohydrates 12g 4% DV; | fat 24g 37% DV; | cholesterol 74.9mg 25% DV; | sodium 694.1mg 28% DV.

Wendy's KETO TEX-MEX STUFFED ZUCCHINI BOATS.

Ingredient

- 1 lb ground beef
- 2 tbsp of butter or olive oil
- 1 tsp of salt
- 2 tbsp Tex-Mex seasoning
- 1 tsp of salt
- ½ cup finely chopped fresh cilantro (optional)
- 2 zucchini
- 1 tbsp olive oil
- 1¼ cups shredded cheese
- 7 oz. Lettuce Lettuce

- 4 tbsp olive oil
- ½ tbsp red wine vinegar or white vinegar 5 percent
- Salt and pepper

Instructions

1. Preheat your oven to 400°F (200°C).

2. Lengthwise, cut each zucchini in half and extract the seeds. Sprinkle with salt and let sit for 10 minutes.

3. Brown the ground meat in olive oil in a frying pan while the zucchini is sitting. Incorporate salt and Tex-Mex seasoning. Let it cook until most of the liquid has evaporated.

4. Blot off the drops of liquid with paper towels. Place the halves in a greased baking dish.

5. Mix a third of the cheese into the ground beef. Add finely-chopped cilantro (optional).

6. Divide the mixture of ground beef and cheese equally between the zucchini vessels. Sprinkle on top of the leftover cheese. Bake for 20 minutes or until the cheese starts to brown in the oven. Take out the zucchini and allow it to cool down for five minutes.

7. In a simple vinaigrette, combine the oil, vinegar, salt, and pepper together. The salad is prepared and eaten alongside the zucchini ferry.

Nutrition Facts

Per Serving: 559 calories; protein 41.8g 84% DV; | carbohydrates 40.8g 13% DV; | fat 25.7g 40% DV; | cholesterol 97.1mg 32% DV; | sodium 690.8mg 28% DV.

Arby's OMELET KETO PIZZA

Ingredients
Crust

- Four eggs
- 5 oz. Cheese mozzarella, shredded
- 4 tbsp of cream cheese
- 1/4 tsp of salt
- 1 tsp powder with garlic
- Topping With
- 3 cups of tomato sauce
- Six oz. Cheese mozzarella, shredded
- 2 tsp of oregano dried

Instructions

1. Preheat the oven to 400 ° F (200 ° C).
2. Begin the crust by creating it. Crack the eggs and add the remaining ingredients to a medium-sized dish. To mix, give it a nice stir.
3. Line a pie plate with parchment paper (a normal-sized pie plate is large enough for two parts) or some other oven-proof dish (crumple the sheet until you flatten it out so that it sits down faster). Pour in the flour for the pie crust. Using a spatula, spread it out

uniformly. Bake for 15 minutes in the oven before the crust of the pizza is brown.

4. Using the backside of a spoon to scatter tomato sauce onto the crust. Cheese on top.
5. Bake for 10 more minutes, or until the pizza turns golden brown.
6. Sprinkle and serve with oregano.

Nutrition Facts

Per Serving:

336 calories; protein 22g 44% DV; | carbohydrates 8.5g 3% DV; | fat 24.3g 37% DV; | cholesterol 77mg 26% DV; | sodium 638.9mg 26% DV.

Blaze Pizza's KEDOUGH PIZZA 'S SULLIVAN

Ingredients

About the crust

- 1/2 cup of unflavored whey extract protein powder
- 1/2 tsp baking powder
- 1/2 tsp of garlic granulated
- 1/2 tsp of salt
- 1/2 tsp of Italian seasoning
- Three oz. Grated Cheese and Parmesan
- Three oz. Cheese with mozzarella
- Two oz. Cheese with cream cheese
- 4 tablespoons olive oil
- 1 egg

The Toppings

- 1/4 cup of tomato sauce unsweetened
- 8 oz. Cheddar Cheese Shredded
- 1/2 with red bell pepper
- 8 oz. Italian New Sausage
- 1 tbsp new basil chopped

Instructions Approaches

1. Preheat the oven to 190 ° C (375 ° F).

3. In a large mixing cup, add all of the ingredients. The bread is going to be a dense batter rather than a workable bread.

4. With parchment paper, cover a baking sheet or pizza block. To smooth the dough into a 9-inch circular pizza crust, use a wooden spoon or spatula. You can also split the dough into fourths to produce four (if you make 4 servings) 5-inch (13 cm) pizza crusts.

5. Bake for 9 to 12 minutes or until the crust turns golden brown.

6. Remove the crust from the oven, cover with your choice pizza toppings and tomato sauce, or save the crusts for later use.

7. Return it to the oven to bake after you top the pizza, before the toppings are browned, and the cheese is melted.

Nutrition Facts

Per Serving: 170 calories; protein 4.8g 10% DV; | carbohydrates 28.1g 9% DV; | fat 4g 6% DV; | cholesterol mg; | sodium 292.8mg 12% DV.

CHAPTER SEVEN

DESSERT

The Cheesecake Factory's CINNAMON ROLL CHEESECAKE

Ingredients

- for 8 servings
- 16 oz cream cheese, melted
- ½ cup sugar
- ½ cup sour cream
- 1 teaspoon vanilla extract
- 2 chickens
- 1/2 cup of butter, melted
- 1/2 cup of light brown sugar
- 2 tablespoons of cinnamon
- 1 box of refrigerated rolls of cinnamon with frosting

Preparation

1. Preheat the oven to 160 ° C/325 ° F.
2. In a cup beat the cream cheese and sugar until fluffy.
3. Add the vanilla and sour cream and beat until no lumps are left.
4. Add the eggs one at a time, mixing thoroughly with each one. Put aside, just.
5. In another dish, combine the butter, brown

sugar, and cinnamon until thoroughly combined. Put aside, just.

6. In a greased spring-form tray, press all the cinnamon rolls flat until the tray's bottom is filled.
7. Spread the cheesecake batter equally, and apply the butter mixture to the cheesecake batter with a spoonful.
8. Swirl the butter mixture into the cheesecake (try to keep it away from the edges!) using a knife.
9. Bake for 30-35 minutes, until the cheesecake is stable around the edges but still slightly jiggly in the middle.
10. Delete from the oven and cool down.
11. Fill the cinnamon rolls with frosting.
12. Please at least refrigerate for 4 hours.

Nutrition Facts

Per Serving: 372 calories; | protein 6.4g 13% DV; | carbohydrates 45.2g 15% DV; | fat 18.9g 29% DV; | cholesterol 51.4mg 17% DV; | sodium 198mg 8% DV.

California Pizza Kitchen's TOFFEE TILES

Ingredients

For the 15 servings

Toffee-toffee, Toffee-toffee

- 6 tablespoons of salted butter (84 g)
- 3/4 cups of medium brown sugar (165 g),

thinly packed
- 1 teaspoon kosher salt (5 g)
- 10 finely chopped almonds
- The Coatings
- 1 milk chocolate bar
- 1/8 teaspoon of salt from the pink ocean
- 1 tablespoon of butter (14 g)
- For Special Products
- Liquid thermometer
- Parchment-based paper

Preparation

1. Cover the baking tray with parchment paper.
2. In a saucepan, combine the butter, sugar, and salt. Remove before the temperature reaches 260 ° F. from the sun.
3. Sprinkle the sliced almonds into the mixture and thoroughly blend them in.
4. Add the mixture to the baking pan.
5. Place the baking tray in the fridge for 30-45 minutes.
6. The chocolate bar is melted until it is mixed and covered with salt and melted sugar.
7. Slice the toffee from the fridge and divide it into chunks. Then coat it in the melted chocolate mixture.
8. Put the chocolate-covered toffee bits back on the parchment-lined baking tray and hold them in the refrigerator for 15 minutes.

9. Crop the chocolate-covered toffee from the freezer and tray. With a bottle of milk, enjoy yourself!

Nutrition Facts

Per Serving:

226 calories; | protein 1.5g 3% DV; | carbohydrates 20g 7% DV; | fat 16.9g 26% DV; | cholesterol 30.5mg 10% DV; | sodium 101.1mg 4% DV.

Bonefish Grill's CLOUD SUGAR PIE BAR

Ingredients

For twelve servings
- Twenty four graham crackers smashed
- Unsalted butter of 12 teaspoons, melted
- 5 oz of an instant mix of vanilla pudding (145 g)
- 2 1/2 cups of (600 mL) heavy cream
- 1/2 cup (85 g) chocolate candy pieces
- Whipped cream, to be served

Preparation

1. Line the parchment paper with a baking sheet.
2. Mix the graham cracker crumbs and butter in a medium bowl until thoroughly integrated.
3. Pour the crumbs onto the baking sheet that has been prepared and push tightly into an even plate. Transfer to the refrigerator for 1 hour, roughly.

4. Combine the pudding mix and heavy cream in the bowl of a stand mixer fitted with the whisk attachment, and whip until light and fluffy, for around 5 minutes.
5. Spread the pudding and cover with the candy bits over the crust.
6. Cut into 12 bars with a dollop of whipped cream and serve.
7. Enjoy! Enjoy!

Nutrition Facts
Per Serving:291 calories; | protein 4.4g 9% DV; | carbohydrates 45.7g 15% DV; | fat 10.7g 16% DV; | cholesterol 92.6mg 31% DV; | sodium 88.1mg 4% DV.

Maggiano's Little Italy's CHOCO COOKIES CHIP

Ingredients
For fifteen cookies
- 1 cup of brown sugar
- 1 cup of sugar caster
- 1 Amul butter stick
- Two chickens
- 2 teaspoons of an extract of vanilla
- 1 teaspoon powder for baking
- 1/4 teaspoon of salt
- 3 cups of flour Maida
- 1 dark chocolate chip cup
- Butter to grease the pan

Preparation, preparation

1. Combine the brown sugar and caster sugar.
2. Let the butter melt. When paired with the sugars, ensure it is at room temperature.
3. One at a time, add the eggs. Mix thoroughly.
4. Add the essence of vanilla, baking powder, and salt.
5. In batches, incorporate the Maida.
6. Add the chocolate chips now.
7. Mix well for all the ingredients.
8. Oven for 10 minutes, preheat at 300 ° F (150 ° C).
9. In the meantime, by adding butter, prepare the baking pan.
10. Break the dough into small balls, leaving 11/2-2 inch holes between the dough.
11. For 15-17 minutes, bake.
12. Take the tray out until the timer goes off and let the cookies cool on it; they could get trapped in the tray.

Nutrition Facts

Per Serving:

125 calories; | protein 1.5g 3% DV; | carbohydrates 15.5g 5% DV; fat 7.1g 11% DV; | cholesterol 17.9mg 6% DV; | sodium 63.1mg 3% DV.

Shake Shack's <u>LIGHT SWEET CAKE OF POTATO</u>

Ingredients

For eight servings

- 1 1/2 cups flour (185 g)
- 1/2 cup of wheat flour (65 g)
- 2 bread powder teaspoons
- 1/2 teaspoon of baking soda
- 1 cinnamon teaspoon
- 1/8 teaspoon of salt
- 1/4 teaspoon of ginger
- Two chickens
- 1/2 teaspoon vanilla vanilla
- 1/2 cup (120 mL) milk
- 1/4 cup (60 mL) oil
- 2/3 cup sugar (135 g)
- 2 tablespoons of honey
- 1 cup (260 g) of sweet potato purée

For serving, peanut butter (optional)

Preparation

1. Then, combine the dry ingredients separately with the wet ingredients.
2. Mix them then.
3. Pour into a pan of the loaf
4. Bake for 50 minutes to 1 hour at 350 ° F (180 ° C) in the oven.
5. Optional: with peanut butter, serve it.

Nutrition Facts

Per Serving:

291 calories; | protein 4.4g 9% DV; | carbohydrates 45.7g 15% DV; | fat 10.7g 16% DV; cholesterol 92.6mg 31% DV; | sodium 88.1mg 4% DV.

RECIPES without MEAT: KETO DIET

Panda Express's The Warm Wings

Ingredients

For a serving of 1

- 6 wings of chicken
- Salt, for taste
- Pepper, to taste
- Spray with olive oil
- 4 tablespoons of salted butter
- Worcestershire sauce 1 splash
- 5 teaspoons of Frank's Red Hot Initial

Preparation

1. Salt and wings with pepper.
2. Spray them with olive oil so that they do not bind together.
3. Put the chicken wings in the fryer for 10 minutes at 350 ° F (175 ° C). Uh. Flip. Air fry for an extra 10 minutes.
4. Let the butter melt. Add Worcestershire and red-hot Frank.
5. In the sauce, drink the chicken.

Nutrition Facts

Per Serving:

523 calories; | protein 17.2g 34% DV; | carbohydrates 33.5g 11% DV; | fat 35.1g 54% DV; | cholesterol 45.8mg 15% DV; | sodium 1003.8mg 40% DV.

Panda Express's BEEF STEW HEARTY CROCK-POT

Ingredients

For eight servings

- 1 Mccormick ® beef stew seasoning packet
- Bottle of 1 v8 juice (46 oz)
- 4 celeries, thinly sliced
- 1 Onion Vidalia, sliced into slices
- 1 (18 oz) carrot bag
- Six red potatoes, cut into 1/8 of each piece,
- 1 1/2 lb of stewed (680 g) beef meat

Preparation

1. Turn on the slow cooker's high setting to
2. Put the stewed meat in the slow cooker and 2/3 of the baby carrots and the sliced celery.
3. Set one half of the onion aside. Dice them and add the other half to the Crock-Pot. Have some potatoes attached.
4. In a big pot, mix the 3 cups of V8 juice and the seasoning package. Add the liquid to the slow cooker.

5. With a large cooking spoon, stir the stew slowly until it is relatively mixed.
6. Cook for 2.5 hours or until you have soft potatoes and carrots.

Nutrition Facts

Per Serving:

201 calories; | protein 14.3g 29% DV; | carbohydrates 27.4g 9% DV; | fat 4.5g 7% DV; cholesterol 22.5mg 8% DV; | sodium 512.3mg 21% DV.

<u>Taco Bell's SIMPLE SAUSAGE WITH PASTA</u>

Ingredients

Four dinners, four dinners
Olive oil, for tasting,

- 1 onion, thinly sliced
- 4 sausage halves
- 1/2 cup flakes of red pepper
- 1/2 Teaspoon of Black Pepper
- 3 crushed tomatoes cans
- 4 cloves of garlic, minced
- 1 Teaspoon of oregano
- 1 tablespoon of dry basil, divided, plus one teaspoon
- 1/2 Bag for Penne pasta
- 1/6 block parmesan cheese

Preparation

1. Heat a 2-liter pot and add a little bit of olive

oil to it. Place the onion and sausage in the oven when the oven is warmed up. Apply red pepper flakes and black pepper.

2. Pour in the crushed tomatoes in 3 cans until the sausage is seared. Pour in 1/2 cup of water. Add some cloves of ground garlic. Oregano is applied, along with one tablespoon of basil. Let it cook under low pressure for an hour and a half.

3. In a different pot, heat some water to a quick boil. Add the penne-pasta. Until it is baked, strain the pasta.

4. In a small tub, serve both the pasta and sauce with half a sausage and finish with the parmesan and basil.

Nutrition Facts

Per Serving:

201 calories; | protein 14.3g 29% DV; | carbohydrates 27.4g 9% DV; | fat 4.5g 7% DV; | cholesterol 22.5mg 8% DV; | sodium 512.3mg 21% DV.

Arby's EASY ENCHILADAS FOR CHICKEN CHICKENS

Ingredients

Holding five servings

- 1 chicken cup, shredded (100 g)
- 1/4 Cup of Maize (40 g)
- 1/2 cup (50 g) shredded cheese

- 1 can of enchilada sauce, 19 ounces (535 grams)
- 5 tortillas

Preparation

1. Heat your oven to 350 ° F (180 ° C).
2. Mix chicken, maize, enchilada (leave 1/4 cup for top and base) sauce, and 1/4 cup (25 G) cheese in a dish.
3. Put a thin layer of enchilada sauce in a pan.
4. Put a thin film of enchilada sauce on top of the pan.
5. Dip the tortilla on a tray with the enchilada sauce until it gets soaked. Cover with the roll and chicken mixture. Set the pan in place.
6. With the leftover cheese and enchilada sauce, coat the completed enchiladas.
7. Bake until cheese is melted for 15 minutes.
8. Enjoy! Enjoy! Enjoy! Enjoy!

Nutrition Facts

Per Serving:

829 calories; | protein 45.2g 90% DV; | carbohydrates 58.4g 19% DV; | fat 46.9g 72% DV; | cholesterol 145.8mg 49% DV; | sodium 2485.6mg 99% DV.

Arby's BACON AVOCADO SALAD CAESAR SALAD CAESAR

Ingredients

For two servings,

- 1 head of Roman lettuce
- 4 fried and crumbled bacon strips
- 1 avocado, chopped-up
- 1/2 cup of crouton (15 g)
- 1/2 cup parmesan shaved cheese (55 g), add more to serve
- 1/4 cup Caesar dressing (60 g)

Preparation

1. Break the lettuce into pieces of around 1 inch (2 1/2 cm), then transfer to a large salad bowl.
2. Tie bacon, avocado, croutons, cheese, and dressing together and combine until combined uniformly.
3. On top of the extra parmesan, serve.
4. Enjoy! Enjoy! Enjoy! Enjoy!

Nutrition Facts

Per Serving:

745 calories; | protein 20.6g 41% DV; carbohydrates 70.7g 23% DV; | fat 42.1g 65% DV; cholesterol 30.1mg 10% DV; | sodium 1554mg 62% DV.

Jack in the Box's BEEF BURGERS WITH SAUCE WITH CREAMY MUSHROOM

Ingredients

For two servings,

- 2 patties of ground beef

- 2 burger buns
- 7 oz (200 g) heavy cream
- 4 cups (960 mL) white wine
- 1 red, diced onion
- 3 cups of fungi (250 g)
- 2 black figs, cut
- Combination of salt and pepper, to taste

Preparation

1. For the sauce: In a saucepan, melt olive oil over medium heat. Attach the red onion and fry for about 1-2 minutes. Stir in the cut mushrooms and sauté for 2-3 more minutes. With salt, season.
2. To deglaze the mushrooms, add white wine and milk. Let the mixture boil for five minutes.
3. For the burgers: steam the patties until the buns are cooked through and toast on the BBQ or stovetop.
4. Cut any figs.
5. Place the mushroom sauce and sliced fig on top of the patties and put in the buns.

Nutrition Facts

Per Serving:

952 calories; | protein 62.7g 125% DV; | carbohydrates 39.5g 13% DV; | fat 61.3g 94% DV; | cholesterol 195.5mg 65% DV; sodium 1063.9mg 43% DV.

Carol Winehouse's CHICKEN FROM ROAST TARRAGON CHICKEN

Ingredients

Holding five servings
- 1/4 cup of butter (115 g), split
- 5 thin, peeled sweet potatoes
- 4 celery stalks
- 2 big sweet onions
- 5 little sweet red peppers
- 5 tiny yellow peppers
- 2 tablespoons of olive oil
- 1 tablespoon red pepper flakes
- 2 teaspoons of garlic powder
- 3 teaspoons of fresh tarragon, sliced
- 1 whole chicken, 2 kg (5 pounds)
- Salt, for taste
- Pepper, to taste
- 1 cup stock of chicken (240 mL), unsalted
- 1 teaspoon of cayenne pepper ground

Preparation

1. Using some of the butter to oil the large roasting pan well.
2. Preheat the oven to 375 ° F (190 ° C).
3. Chop all the vegetables roughly (they might cook too well or get mushy if you don't).
4. In a big tub, mix all the vegetables. Sprinkle with one tablespoon of tarragon, olive oil, garlic powder, and pepper flakes. Put aside,

just.

5. Pat the chicken dry, making sure that the chicken leaves no innards. To the chicken's interior, add one tablespoon of tarragon and a pinch of salt and pepper.

6. Carefully blend the remaining butter and place the tarragon on top of the breasts under the chicken's skin.

7. Place a small oven-safe gratin or shelf at the bottom of the roasting pan, then pour your mixed vegetables in. Apply it with half a cup of chicken stock.

8. On top of the shelf put the chicken, so it sits above the stock and vegetables.

9. Aluminum foil or lid cover. Place in the oven, with 1/2 cup of chicken stock as desired, to keep the vegetables moist but not submerged. Cook 2 hours of chicken (cooking times vary according to the chicken and oven configuration). Remove it from the oven and break the cover when the chicken is almost cooked, using ground cayenne pepper and salt to sprinkle.

10. To brown, bring the chicken back in the oven for 10-15 minutes.

11. Enjoy! Enjoy! Enjoy! Enjoy!

Nutrition Facts

Per Serving: 316 calories; | protein 56.6g 113% DV; | carbohydrates 2.9g 1% DV; fat 7g 11% DV; | cholesterol 151.8mg 51% DV; | sodium 1280.5mg 51% DV.

Jack in the Box's BBQ CHICKEN POPCORN BREADED

Ingredients
Four dinners, four dinners
- 2 boneless, skinless chicken breasts
- 1 tablespoon of hot sauce
- For 1 cup, BBQ sauce, plus more to serve
- 1 tablespoon sauce peri-peri
- 1 tablespoon lemon juice
- 1 tablespoon of smoked paprika
- 1 tablespoon chili powder
- 1 tablespoon brown sugar
- 2 teaspoons of bbq seasoning, breakage
- 3 tablespoons of coconut oil;
- 1/3 cup of popcorn, yellow (40 g)
- 1 melted butter tablespoon
- 1 bbq chips are going to

Preparation
1. Clean and channel the bosoms of chicken.
2. Mix the hot sauce, BBQ sauce, peri-peri sauce, and lemon juice in a medium dish.
3. Combine the smoked paprika, bean stew powder, earthy colored sugar, and half the BBQ preparation in another bowl of a similar size.
4. Drizzle the chicken bosoms with the wet mix, making a point of having the two sides.
5. Sprinkle on the chicken bosoms with the dry

mix, making a point of having the two sides.

6. In the cooler, marinate the chicken breasts for 4 hours.

7. Preheat the broiler to 425 ° F (220 ° C) after 4 hours or anywhere in the vicinity.

8. Place the enormous pan over medium-high heat. In the pan, soften the coconut oil. In the pot, put 3 or 4 bits of popcorn. Include the remainder of the pieces as they pop, place on the lid, and extract the warmth. Place it back on the burner after 30 seconds or so. Shake yourself periodically. Delete from the heat if the popping reduces to like clockwork.

9. On the kernels, pour the softened margarine and mix to get the kernels' whole. Include the remainder of the preparation of the BBQ, blending to get the whole popcorn.

10. Grind 2/3 of the popcorn alongside the chips from the BBQ. Sprinkle this over the chicken bosoms that are marinated, attempting to get the two sides. The marinade should accompany the popcorn morsels.

11. For 18-20 minutes, roast the chicken. When packed, show the rest of the popcorn and the BBQ sauce with the rest.

12. Enjoy! Enjoy!

Nutrition Facts

Per Serving: 238 calories; | protein 3.4g 7% DV; | carbohydrates 21.9g 7% DV; | fat 16.3g 25% DV; |

cholesterol mg; | sodium 387.6mg 16% DV.

KFC's CHICKEN PEPPER

Ingredients

Six meals with six meals

- Three teaspoons of oil
- 1 big onion, sliced
- 1 teaspoon of garlic ginger adhesive
- Three green chiles
- 1/2 teaspoon of turmeric powder
- 2 tablespoons of dark peppercorn
- 1 tomato giant, hacked
- 2 lb (1 kg) chicken
- 1 gigantic potato, cut into bits
- Salt, for taste

Preparation

1. In a hot container, with oil included. Have the onion and sauté until soft earthy colored after the oil warms up.
2. Ginger-garlic glue and chilies are applied and sautéed for a second.
3. Break the peppercorns and sauté well in the turmeric powder.
4. Attach the tomato and let it cook until it turns tender and delicate.
5. Now, put the chicken in and blend everything. Spread the bowl, set it on low heat, and cook until half of the chicken is cooked. (This is an ideal chance to include

the potato if it is used).

6. Cover and cook until finished, and dry all the chicken juices. There should be no water added to this dish as the chicken cooks with salt in its juices.
7. Enjoy! Enjoy!

Nutrition Facts

Per Serving: 234 calories; | protein 16.7g 33% DV; | carbohydrates 21.2g 7% DV; fat 9.4g 14% DV; | cholesterol 52.8mg 18% DV; | sodium 1252.5mg 50% DV.

McDonald's ONE-POT CHICKEN BAKEE FIERY ONE-POT

Ingredients

For four meals

- McCormick ® Zesty Spice Mix 2 teaspoons, partitioned
- 1 tablespoon right salt, removed, one tablespoon genuine salt
- 1/2 teaspoon of dark pepper freshly ground
- 1 pound boneless, skinless thighs of chicken (455 g)
- 1 tablespoon of vegetable oil
- 2 tablespoons of margarine without salt
- 1 yellow, medium onion, diced
- 1 medium red, cultivated and chopped ringer pepper
- 3 garlic cloves, minced
- 2 cups of white long-grain rice (400 g,

basmati or jasmine, for example)
- 4 cups stock of chicken (960 mL)
- 1 lemon, cut
- New basil, big little cluster, meagerly sliced

Preparation

1. Preheat the broiler to a temperature of 190 ° C (375 ° F)
2. Combine one tablespoon of Zesty's zest blend, one teaspoon of salt, and pepper in a shallow cup. Cover each chicken piece evenly with the mixture to cook. Place yourself in a comfortable spot.
3. Heat the vegetable oil in a 6-quart Dutch oven over medium-high heat. Burn the chicken on either side for 2-3 minutes, operating in clumps, before a brilliant earthy colored covering structure is available. Move the chicken to a plate and place the chicken in a safe place.
4. Decrease the heat to medium. Spread, onion, and garlic included. Once the onion is translucent and fragrant, cook for 2 minutes.
5. Attach the rice and the remaining tablespoon of the Zesty flavor blend, the ringer pepper, and the margarine and aromatic mixture to coat. To deglaze the pot, pour in the stock and mix. Have two teaspoons of salt for your visit. Place it in a tiny bubble and cook for about 2 minutes.
6. Arrange the bits of chicken on the rice head. They can slightly sink into the stock. That is,

though, okay.

7. Cover and move the Dutch broiler to the burner. Prepare for 35 minutes until the rice is baked, though not fluffy, and the chicken's temperature exceeds 165 ?? F (75 ?? C).

8. From the oven, extract the chicken. Crush the juice into the rice from the lemon half and cushion with a fork, allowing steam to get away and avoid cooking further.

9. Switch to plates the rice and chicken and top with fresh basil. Cut the remaining half of the lemon into wedges, then serve as an afterthought.

10. Enjoy! Enjoy!

Nutrition Facts

Per Serving:

515 calories; | protein 42.5g 85% DV; | carbohydrates 53.7g 17% DV; | fat 12.9g 20% DV; | cholesterol 87.2mg 29% DV; | sodium 757.9mg 30% DV.

Baja Fresh's QUINOA RICE CAKES RICE CAKES

Ingredients

- 2 packets of radical natural quinoa seeds and earthy flavored garlic rice
- 3/4 cup zucchini (115 g), destroyed, water crushed out by overabundance
- 2 teaspoons of fresh parsley, minced

- 1 squeeze of lemon, and zing
- 1 dried oregano teaspoon
- 1 teaspoon of ground cilantro
- 1/2 teaspoon paprika
- 3 whisked eggs
- 2/3 cup (75 g) whole-wheat breadcrumbs
- 1/4 cup of feta cheddar, disintegrated (25 g)
- 1/4 cup (60 mL) olive oil
- Cherry tomatoes, for embellishment,
- Olive kalamata, for embellishment

Instructions

1. To make a marinade, combine the garlic, salt, pepper, olive oil, and lemon juice.
2. In the mixture, toss the chicken and let it marinate for 15-20 minutes.
3. The bundles of Organic Quinoa Seeds of Change and Brown Rice with Garlic are cut open, so the opening is about 2 inches (5 cm) wide.
4. 90-second microwave packets. Place the material into a bowl at that point.
5. Apart from the olive oil, add the rest of the rice cake fixings and mix well.
6. In a food processor, extract about 1/3 of the mix and heartbeat it well.
7. Back in the remainder of the mix, add the beat quinoa and join well.
8. Take around 1/3 cup (45 g) of quinoa mix to form quinoa cakes and shape into a small patty using your hands. For the rest of the

quinoa mix, Rehash.

9. In a big pan, melt the olive oil. Cook the quinoa cakes on either side for 3-4 minutes until they are brilliantly earthy. Eliminate from skillet.

10. In a different skillet, heat a shower of olive oil. Burn two sides of marinated chicken.

11. Cover the dish with a top to hold the chicken cooked until the temperature reaches 165oF (75oFC).

12. Shift the chicken and let it rest for 5 minutes on a cutting board.

13. Break the chicken into thin cuts.

14. Placed a couple of pieces of chicken on a quinoa cake for the party.

15. Garnish the tomatoes with them. Set a second quinoa cake on top at that stage to frame a sandwich.

16. Enjoy! Enjoy!

Nutrition Facts

Per Serving:

720 calories; | protein 48.5g 82% DV; | carbohydrates 94.7g 17% DV; | fat 12.9g 20% DV; cholesterol 87.2mg 29% DV; | sodium 757.9mg 30% DV.

CHAPTER EIGHT

SNACKS

Dominos' PIZZA WITH ARTICHOKES LOW-CARB CAULIFLOWER

Ingredients

Garnishes

Pureed tomatoes 2 tbsp

- Two oz. Cheddar Destroyed
- 1 tbsp of dried oregano or basil dried
- Two oz. Cheddar mozzarella
- Two oz. Artichokes in a can, cut into wedges
- 1 clove of garlic, meagerly cut (discretionary)
- 41/4 oz. Cheddar Destroyed
- 41/4 oz. Cauliflower soil
- Two chickens
- 1/2 tsp of salt

Instructions

1. Preheat the broiler at 180 ° C (350 ° F). Mash the cauliflower in a food processor or in a grater. Gather the ruined cheddar and eggs in a bowl and combine well into a single unit.

2. Using a spatula, spread meagerly on a planning sheet fixed with material tape, 11

inches (28 cm) in diameter. Prepare for about 20 minutes or until a warm sound has turned around, but similar to that.

3. Remove it from the oven. The pureed tomatoes are laid out, and the cheddar top is used. Cover with discretionary garlic and artichokes. Sprinkle on top of oregano/basil.

4. Elevate the temperature to 210 ° C (420 ° F) and cook the pizza for another 5-10 minutes.

Yeah, Tip!

You can buy pureed tomatoes or make your tomatoes. Tomato glue damaged by a little water or a thinly slashed tomato may also be used. It is too tasty for Ajvar relish or red tomato pesto.

Nutrition Facts

Per Serving:

704 calories; | protein 36.2g 72% DV; | carbohydrates 30.6g 10% DV; | fat 51.3g 79% DV; cholesterol 225.9mg 75% DV; | sodium 2040.2mg 82% DV.

Blaze Pizza's SMALL PIZZAS

Ingredients

Outside
- 3 eggs
- 5 ounces of mayonnaise
- 3 tbsp of flour of coconut
- 1 tsp powder preparation
- 1/2 tsp of salt

- 1/2 tsp powder of onion
- 1 tablespoon of olive oil

Instructions

- 8 tablespoons of tomato glue or green pesto or cheddar cream
- 1 Tsp of salt from the ocean
- 1/4 tsp dark pepper field
- 8 oz. Destroyed cheddar mozzarella
- Two oz. Ground cheddar parmesan
- 1 tablespoon of olive oil
- 12 olives or shrimp or cherry tomatoes, or chorizo air-dried

Food

Instructions

1. Whisk together in a cup of eggs and mayonnaise. Blend individually dried fixings and overlap them in the eggs. For a quick hitter, mix. Let yourself wait for two or three minutes.

2. In a hot skillet with grease, add the hitter. It should be 8-10 outside, around 3 inches (8 cm) in the distance.

3. On either hand, fry for a moment before genius. Using the broiler's sear setup, preheat a stove to 400 ° F (200 ° C). Spot the outside on a planning sheet fixed with content tape.

4. When you need a red, green, or white pizza, apply a tomato glue, pesto, or cream cheddar layer. Or, on the other hand, as we have done, mix!

5. Add corrections to the vote. Sprinkle on top with salt, pepper, and basil or oregano. Add the cheddar and sprinkle the top with olive oil.

6. Bake for 5-10 minutes in the oven or until the cheddar is dissolved, and the pizzas transform to a familiar sound. Serve immediately!

Tip

Any repair for the tiny pizzas can be used. We've chosen a mix of seafood, beef, and vegan choices. Fried ham, bacon, and tuna are other pleasant choices. By using green ringer peppers, stew peppers, or artichoke hearts, you could even make the green pizzas "greener." Onion and garlic are also acceptable for these!

A mix of Mozzarella and Parmesan cheddar is perfect for cheddar, but you can also choose anything interesting. If you prefer more delicious cheeses, blue cheddar, feta cheddar, or goat cheddar would have an exceptional taste expansion.

Nutrition Facts

Per Serving:

704 calories; | protein 36.2g 72% DV; | carbohydrates 30.6g 10% DV; | fat 51.3g 79% DV; | cholesterol 225.9mg 75% DV; | sodium 2040.2mg 82% DV.

Blaze Pizza's OF BARBECUED FLATBREAD

Ingredients

Flatbread

- 1 cup of flour of coconut
- 3 tbsp powder of ground psyllium husk
- 1/2 tsp of heating powder
- 11/2 tsp of salt
- 1 tsp of dark pepper soil
- 4 tablespoons olive oil or coconut oil
- 2 cups of water, hot but not bubbling,
- Garnishes Garnishes
- 10 oz. Cheddar's New Mozzarella
- Six oz. Tomatoes with Cherry Tomatoes
- 2 tbsp of fresh basil
- 2 tablespoons olive oil
- 1 salt squeeze
- 1 dark pepper ground squeeze

Subsistence

Instructions

1. With the cover off, preheat the barbecue for 20-30 minutes at low warmth.
2. Mix the dry components of the flatbread mixture in a dish. Consolidate totally.
3. Olive oil and half of the boiling water should be added. Blend in and consolidate well with a spoon. For a few minutes, blend. Check the accuracy at that point. Remove some more coconut flour on the off chance that the mixture is excessively clingy. Get more water, on the off chance that the batter isn't sticky enough. With your hands, form one ball for each pizza. It shouldn't be messy.
4. For straightening any batter ball between

two sheets of material paper, use a moving screw. In any case, the pizzas must be 1/2-inch (1 cm) wide.

5. Use a paper towel to grease the barbecue with some olive oil to make sure the pizzas are not oily.

6. Brush with olive oil every pizza in order to coat the entire oil board. Flip your palm over the pie and fine-tune it with a slick side down on the barbecue. Rehash for the next pizza. Five minutes on both sides, near cover and grill. Don't feed unbelievably closely just.

7. Brush the pizza's head and flip for a few moments to barbecue the other side, too.

8. Remove from the broil and cover with mozzarella, sliced tomatoes, and fresh basil for each pizza.

9. With the top close, put the pizzas back on the flame broil and barbecue for 5-7 additional minutes.

10. Remove and season with pepper and salt. Use olive oil to sprinkle.

11. No planning for a barbecue

12. Preheat your broiler up to 175 ° C (350 ° F).

13. Shift the straightened pizza mixture onto a heating sheet fixed with material paper after you're done with Step 4. Heat up without the fixings for 25 minutes.

14. Eliminate the garnishes from the broiler, fire for an extra 10 minutes at that stage until

the edges have the right tone and the cheddar has liquefied.

Tips

Do not hesitate to zest up the flatbread batter with additional flavors for even more taste. Garlic powder, oregano, or red pepper drops make the base hull pizza-style even more celestial.

The sponginess of coconut flour and psyllium husk, depending on what brand you buy, varies a significant deal. This ensures that steadily including the heated water before you achieve the perfect consistency is best. Start with a 3/4 cup and, if necessary, have more when you go.

To preserve the fluid, add even more coconut flour if you have added an extra amount of water and the batter is clingy. If the batter is not sufficiently moist, add more water.

Nutrition Facts

Per Serving:

793 calories; protein 48.2g 71% DV; carbohydrates 34.6g 19% DV; fat 58.3g 79% DV; cholesterol 225.9mg 75% DV; sodium 2040.2mg 82% DV.

KETO MEAT LOVERS PIE IDEAS TOPPING

KFC's BASE SAUCES KETO MEAT LOVERS PIZZA

Tomato glue (check for no sugar added)
Pesto
 Tapenade of olives

PIZZA-MEATS KETO MEAT LOVERS

Choose the least-handled, most notable meat substance for all foods and meat that has not been returned to starch, nectar, wheat, or grains. Pick meat off the bone and stop the heart that is pre-shaped.

- Ham-off of the bone
- Bacon
- Pepperoni
- Salami
- Biersticks
- Mince / ground / chicken / pork hamburger
- Diced Frankfurter-Diced
- Smoked chicken
- Pastrami
- Chorizo

KETO MEAT LOVERS PIZZA-CHEESESESES LOVERS

- Mozzarella
- Parmesan
- Cheddar

- Mild Mild
- Colby
- Edam
- Blue cheddar
- Camembert
- Brief
- Ricotta
- Grúyere
- Cheddar goats (feta)

HERBS AND SPICES KETO MEAT LOVERS PIZZA

- Chilli
- Rosemary
- Oregano
- Thyme

VEGETABLES AND GREENERY KETO MEAT LOVERS PIZZA

- Onions thinly sliced
- Garlic
- Basil
- Onions of spring
- Champignons
- Chives
- Mint
- Bell peppers
- Olives
- Tomatoes sun-dried

- Avocado
- Fennel

Ingredients

The base of Fat Head Pizza

- The cheapest is 170 g pre-destructed / ground cheddar mozzarella or Edam / mellow cheddar mozzarella.
- 85 g almond feast/flour * see beneath notes
- 2 tbsp of cheddar cream
- 1 egg
- pinch salt to taste
- Herbs and flavors * see above formula notes
- Meat and garnish selection * I use ham, pepperoni, and bier sticks

The Rules

1. In a microwaveable dish, combine the destroyed/grounded cheddar and almond flour/feast (or coconut flour if used). For an instant, including the cream cheddar-microwave on HIGH.
2. Stir, then stir for an additional 30 seconds on HIGH.
3. Combine the egg, salt, spices, flavors or flavorings, and blend gently.
4. Place two pieces of heating material/paper in the middle and fold into the form of a roundabout pizza (see images here). Eliminate the top paper/material planning.
5. To ensure it cooks evenly, makes fork gaps

anywhere on the Fat Head pizza foundation.

6. Slide the pizza-based preparation paper/material on a heating plate (treat plate) or pizza block, ready for 12-15 minutes at 220C/425F, or until earthy.

7. If the top is baked, turn the pizza over (to prepare paper/material) to make the base completely solid and sturdy.

8. Remove from the broiler until cooked and add all the meat and fixings you need. Ensure that any beef is grilled now, as it just returns to warmth and softens the cheddar in the broiler this time—Re-prepare for 5 minutes at 220C/425F.

Nutrition Facts

Per Serving: | 403 calories; | protein 46.9g 72% DV; | carbohydrates 38.6g 13% DV; | fat 51.3g 79% DV; | cholesterol 225.9mg 75% DV; | sodium 2040.2mg 82% DV.

Dominos' LOW-CARB KETO-ACCOMMODATING PIZZA ACCOMMODATING

Ingredients

- 12 ounces of ruined cheddar mozzarella
- Cheddar 2 ounces milk

- 1 2/3 cup (200 g) of finely ground white almond flour, in addition to extra white almond flour for spraying.

- 2 tablespoons of coconut flour (12 g)

- 2 teaspoons for powder preparation

- 2 eggs at room temperature (100 g, weighed out of the shell), beaten

- Decision Fixings (unsweetened pureed tomatoes, more cheddar destroyed)

Instructions

Preheat to 350 ° F your stove. While it preheats, spot a pizza stone or toppled rimmed preparation board in the broiler.

Place the cream cheddar in a medium pot and melt over low heat. Include the mozzarella in two parts, combining delicately until smooth and liquefied. Include around a third of the almond flour, the coconut flour, the preparation powder, and blend until the softened cheddar retains the flour with a silicone spatula. Include the majority of the almond flour and blend to combine. Turn the heating off as the fixings appear to brown in the dish. Mix and press the mixture with the spatula until it is mixed all over. Turn it off on the off possibility that the heat is already on. Apply the eggs to the mixture and combine and press again until the batter's coloring and surface are uniform.

Turn out the mixture carefully floured with almond flour on a bit of material paper and work until smooth. Divide the center of the batter and put one half in a protected spot (spread to prevent it from drying out). Click and reveal the original portion of the mixture into a 12-inch round, lightly sprinkling the batter with more almond flour as it becomes clingy and habitually rotating the batter. To make an edge for the outer sheet, cajole the inner edges into the center. To prevent the mixture from swelling up a lot in the stove, the puncture is achieved with a fork's prongs.

Put the first round in the preheated stove, still on the material pad, on the head of the pizza stone or upset heating sheet, and ready for 6 to 8 minutes or until the mixture no longer sparkles. Eliminate the stove lining. For some time in the future, the parbaked batter will be cooled, sealed tightly, and solidified. Rehash yourself for the remainder of the combination.

Top with unsweetened pureed tomatoes and more demolished cheddar, whenever needed, to keep setting up the pizza. Return the pizza to the broiler and cook until the sides are brilliantly earthy. The top of the cheddar is softened (approximately ten more minutes) before cutting and serving; cool quickly.

Nutrition data is per cut (with eight stakes for each exterior, without garnishes in mind). Using the adding machine at Cronometer.com, it is offered as a kindness; moreover, values are conjectured and fluctuate based on natural circumstances, including the particular brands of products used between various parts.

Nutrition Facts

Per Serving:

263 calories; | protein 12.2g 24% DV; | carbohydrates 22.9g 7% DV; | fat 13.6g 21% DV; | cholesterol 23.4mg 8% DV; | sodium 759.1mg 30% DV.

CONCLUSION

The Ketogenic diet is a fruitful health improvement plan. It uses high fat and low sugar fixings to consume fat rather than glucose. Numerous individuals know about the Atkins diet, yet the Keto plan limits carbs significantly more.

Since we are encircled by drive-through joints and handled dinners, it tends to be a test to dodge carb-rich nourishments, yet legitimate arranging can help.

Plan menus and snacks, in any event, seven days early, so you aren't gotten with just high carb supper decisions. Examination Keto plans on the web; there are many acceptable ones to browse. Drench yourself in the Keto way of life, locate your preferred plans, and stick with them.

CPSIA information can be obtained
at www.ICGtesting.com
Printed in the USA
LVHW080821161120
671797LV00009B/405

9 781513 670027